OPHTHALMIC OFFICE PROCEDURES

A Step-by-Step Approach

OPHTHALMIC OFFICE PROCEDURES

A Step-by-Step Approach

Kenneth C. Chern, M.D.
Ophthalmic Consultants of Boston
Boston, Massachusetts

Eliot D. Foley, M.D.
Retina Service
Department of Ophthalmology
Boston University
Boston, Massachusetts

Jacqueline T. Koo, M.D., M.P.H.
Cornea, External Disease
Refractive Surgery and Glaucoma Fellow
Minnesota Eye Consultants, P.A.
Minneapolis, Minnesota

Ashok K. Reddy, M.D.
Retina Fellow
Department of Ophthalmology
Cornell University
New York Presbyterian Hospital
New York, New York

Barry V. Sandoval, M.D.
The Eye Institute
Yuma, Arizona

McGraw-Hill
Medical Publishing Division

New York   Chicago   San Francisco   Lisbon   London   Madrid
Mexico City   Milan   New Delhi   San Juan   Seoul
Singapore   Sydney   Toronto

Ophthalmic Office Procedures

Copyright © 2004 by **The McGraw-Hill Companies, Inc.** All rights reserved. Printed in the United States of America. Except as permitted under the United States Copyright Act of 1976, no part of this publication may be reproduced or distributed in any form or by any means, or stored in a data base or retrieval system without the prior written permission of the publisher.

1 2 3 4 5 6 7 8 9 0   DOC DOC   0 9 8 7 6 5 4

ISBN 0-07-140941-6

This book was set in Times Roman by International Typesetting & Composition.
The editors were Darlene Barela Cooke, Marsha Loeb, and Regina Y. Brown.
The production supervisor was Catherine Saggese.
The art was prepared by Timothy C. Hengst.
The index was prepared by Herr's Indexing Service.
RR Donnelly was printer and binder.

This book was printed on acid-free paper.

Library of Congress Cataloging-in-Publication Data
Ophthalmic office procedures / authors, Kenneth C. Chern ... [et al.]; artist, Timothy C. Hengst.—1st ed.
   p. ; cm.
  ISBN 0-07-140941-6
   1. Eye—Surgery—Handbooks, manuals, etc. 2. Eye—Examination—Handbooks, manuals, etc. 3. Ambulatory surgery—Handbooks, manuals, etc. I. Chern, Kenneth C.
  [DNLM: 1. Eye Diseases—surgery—Handbooks. 2. Eye Diseases—surgery—Pictorial Works. 3. Ambulatory Surgical Procedures—methods—Handbooks. 4. Ambulatory Surgical Procedures—methods—Pictorial Works. 5. Diagnostic Techniques, Ophthalmological—Handbooks. 6. Diagnostic Techniques, Ophthalmological—Pictorial Works. WW 39 O625 2004]
RE80.O645 2004
617.7'1—dc22   2003065181

Contents

PART 6   RETINA

Preface

Ophthalmic Office Procedures is a manual intended for practicing ophthalmologists, optometrists, emergency room physicians, residents, and students outlining the steps for eye procedures performed in the emergency room or an office setting. The book is organized by anatomical area including cornea, glaucoma, cataracts/lens, neuro-ophthalmology, oculoplastics, and retina. It also includes a section with procedures that are most common in pediatric patients.

Each procedure follows a specific format with indications for use, a list of the equipment needed to perform the procedure, and detailed step-by-step description of how to actually perform the procedure. Beautifully drawn black and white illustrations, specifically created for the book, accompany each procedure and highlight important perspectives and helpful techniques. Special precautions and post-procedure expectations are discussed.

This reference can assist in preparation for procedures done daily or as a refresher and guide for seldom used minor operations.

We hope that you will find this manual will prove to be a convenient reference and handy guide.

Kenneth C. Chern, M.D.

Part 1

Cornea
and
External Disease

1

Removal of Corneal Foreign Bodies

INDICATIONS

For removal of metallic and other debris from the surface of the cornea or embedded within the anterior corneal stroma. Do not use this technique if there is a full-thickness corneal perforation or laceration.

EQUIPMENT

- Topical anesthetic (proparacaine or tetracaine drops)
- Wire lid speculum
- Cotton swabs
- Bard-Parker #15 blade or Kimura spatula
- Hand-held rotating burr
- Slit lamp or magnifying loupes
- Cycloplegic drop (cyclopentolate or tropicamide)
- Antibiotic ointment (erythromycin or bacitracin)
- Eye patches and tape

TECHNIQUE

1. Assemble the necessary instruments and supplies.
2. Anesthetize the eye with several drops of topical anesthetic (proparacaine or tetracaine drops).
3. Place the lid speculum to hold the lids open, if needed.
4. With magnifying loupes or at the slit lamp, position the patient and locate the foreign body (Fig. 1-1).
5. While stabilizing your hand against the patient's face or on the slit lamp, dislodge the foreign body with the edge of the #15 Bard-Parker blade or blunt spatula at a 45 degree angle to the corneal surface (Fig. 1-2).
6. Remove as much rust or other debris as possible from the cornea by scraping the base of the defect.
7. A diamond burr can be used in a circular motion to remove a rust ring in the adjacent tissue.
8. Remove loose debris and epithelium with a dry cotton swab.
9. Remove the lid speculum.
10. Instill cycloplegic drop and an antibiotic drop.
11. Patch eye with antibiotic ointment. Do not patch if foreign body involves vegetable matter or if an infection is suspected. If epithelial defect is small, topical antibiotic drops without patching may be sufficient.
12. The surface often heals within a day or two.

NOTES

Glass or other inert material that has been covered with corneal epithelium with no infiltration or inflammation does not necessarily need to be removed. If the foreign body is deeply embedded or if full-thickness perforation is suspected, remove the foreign body in the operating room.

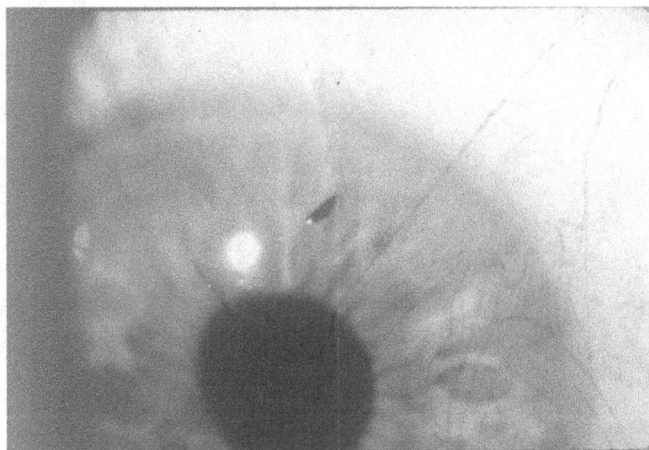

Figure 1-1

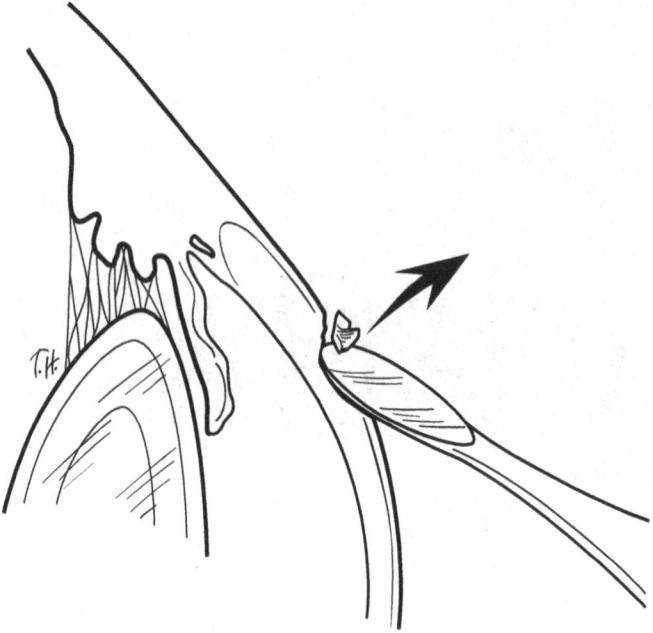

Figure 1-2

2

Anterior Stromal Micropuncture

INDICATIONS

To treat recurrent corneal erosions outside the visual axis after conservative therapy (lubricating ointments, pressure patching, hypertonic saline drops) has failed

EQUIPMENT

- Topical anesthetic drop (proparacaine or tetracaine)
- Wire lid speculum
- Sterile cotton swabs
- 20- or 25-gauge hypodermic needle
- Needle holder
- Bandage contact lens
- Cycloplegic drop
- Antibiotic ointment
- Eye patch

TECHNIQUE

1. Assemble the necessary instruments and supplies.
2. Anesthetize the eye with several drops of topical anesthetic (proparacaine drops).
3. Place the lid speculum to hold the lids open, if needed. Locate area of loose epithelium.
4. Stabilize your hand against the patient's face or on the slit lamp and use the needle to puncture the superficial corneal stroma (Fig. 2-1). If desired, the needle holder can be used to create several bends in the needle to better control the depth of puncture (Fig. 2-2).
5. Remove loose debris and epithelium with a dry cotton swab.
6. Remove the lid speculum.
7. Instill cycloplegic drop.
8. Patch eye with antibiotic ointment. If the epithelial defect is small, topical antibiotic drops without patching may be sufficient. The contact lens may be helpful for improving patient comfort.
9. The surface often heals within a day or two.

PITFALLS

Be watchful of vasovagal episodes elicited by puncture of the cornea with the needle. Avoid stromal puncture in the visual axis since the microscars may scatter light and affect vision.

NOTES

Phototherapeutic keratectomy using the excimer laser is a technique that has been advocated by some as an additional modality for treating this condition. This may be advantageous in patients with erosions in the central cornea.

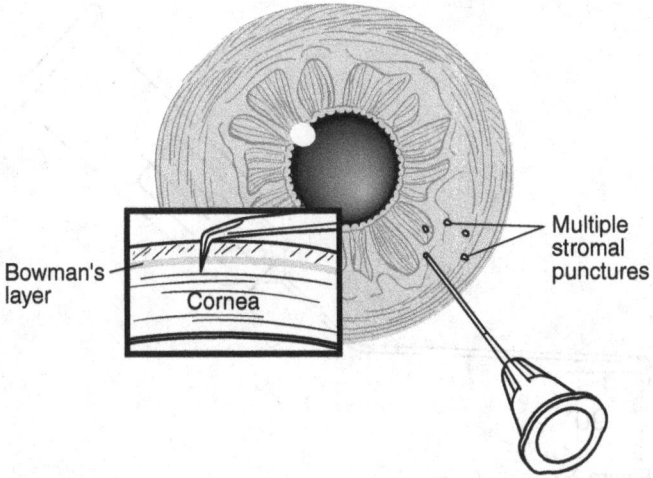

Bowman's layer

Cornea

Multiple stromal punctures

Figure 2-1

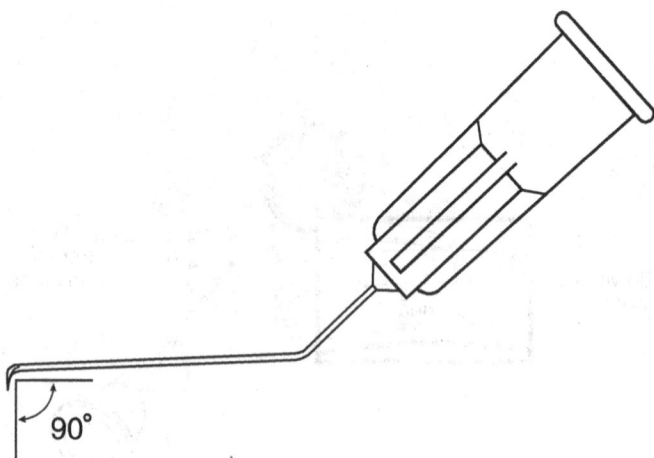

Figure 2-2

3

Corneal Ulcer Scraping and Cultures

INDICATIONS

Suspected infectious corneal ulceration (epithelial defect with stromal thinning) and keratitis. Figure 3-1 shows a whitish corneal infiltrate that was unresponsive to topical antibiotic therapy. Cultures grew fungal colonies.

EQUIPMENT

- Wire lid speculum
- Calcium alginate swabs moistened with sterile saline
- Bard-Parker #15 blade or Kimura spatula
- Glass microscope slides and cytology fixative
- Culture media, warmed to room temperature:
  - Blood agar (2 plates)
  - Chocolate agar
  - Sabouraud agar (fungi)
  - Thioglycollate broth
  - Lowenstein-Jensen slant (mycobacteria)

- Non-nutrient agar with *E. coli* overlay (*Acanthamoeba*)
- Charcoal-yeast agar (*Acanthamoeba*)
- Brain-heart infusion (fungi)
- Viral transport media (viruses)

TECHNIQUE

1. Assemble the necessary instruments and supplies.
2. Anesthetize the eye with several drops of topical anesthetic (proparacaine drops).
3. Place the lid speculum to hold the lids open, if needed.
4. Aggressively swab the base of the ulcer with the calcium-alginate swab and inoculate growth media.
5. Stabilize your hand against the patient's face or against the slit lamp and scrape the base and edges of the ulcer with the surgical blade or spatula (Fig. 3-2).
6. Smear the material onto the slides and apply fixative.
7. Scrape the base of the ulcer to inoculate the culture plates (Fig. 3-3). The culture plate can be divided into quadrants, with the superior quadrants for right and left corneal scrapings and the inferior quadrants for the right and left lid swabs.
8. Remove the lid speculum.
9. If the patient is a contact lens wearer, also culture the contact lens, case, and solutions.

NOTES

Eyelids, conjunctiva, eye dropper tips, contact lenses, and cases may be cultured to provide additional information about possible pathogens.

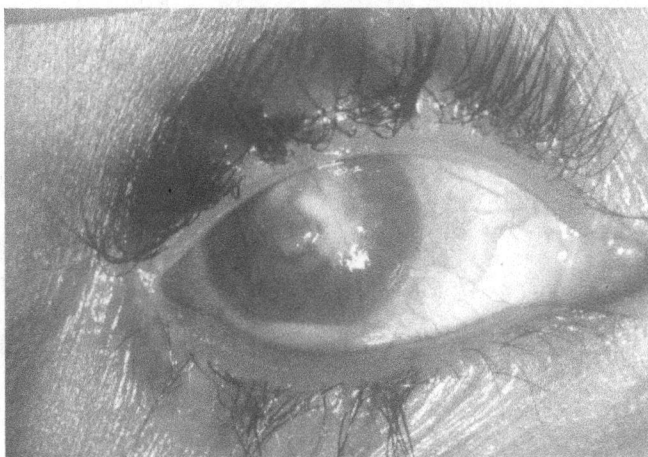

Figure 3-1

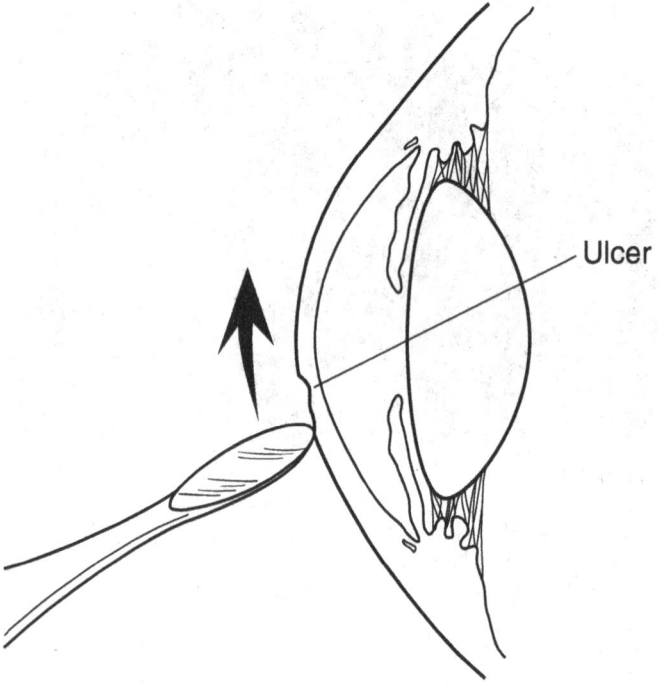

Figure 3-2

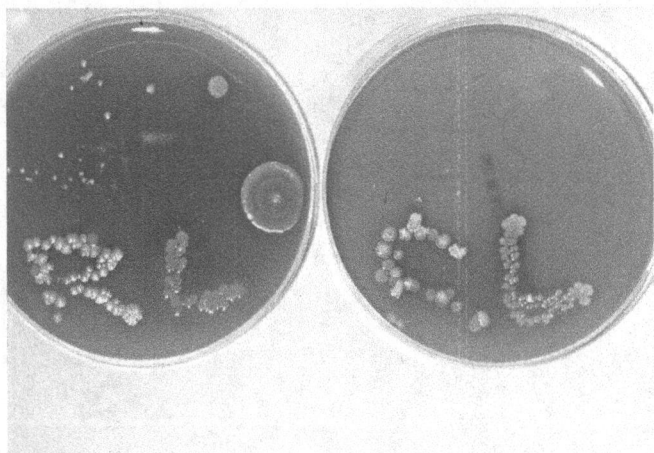

Figure 3-3

4

Anterior Chamber Paracentesis

INDICATIONS

Diagnostic sampling of aqueous fluid (endophthalmitis, ocular lymphoma, etc)

Reduce intraocular pressure (hyphema, central retinal artery occlusion [CRAO], chemical injury, postoperative pressure spike)

Flat anterior chamber reformation

EQUIPMENT

- Proparacaine eye drops
- Broad-spectrum antibiotic eye drops
- 15-Degree supersharp blade
- 1-cc Syringe
- 27- or 30-gauge 5/8-inch hypodermic needle
- BSS (balanced salt solution)

TECHNIQUE

1. Draw up BSS into 1-cc syringe for injection if reforming a flat anterior chamber.
2. Place the patient in the seated position in the examination chair.

3. Instill one drop each of antibiotic and anesthetic into the eye to be tapped.

4. Instruct patient to comfortably rest his or her head in the slit lamp and remain still. If necessary enlist an assistant to help immobilize the patient's head.

5. Hold the supersharp blade parallel to the iris at the limbus (Fig. 4-1a and 4-1b). Insert blade halfway to enter the anterior chamber and withdraw.

6. Hold the syringe with the 30-gauge 5/8-inch hypodermic needle attached between the thumb and middle finger, resting the index finger against the plunger ready to aspirate or inject as required. Rest the other fingers against the forehead strap of the slit lamp.

7. Bring the tip of the needle to the cornea at the stab site. Avoid the cilia (eyelashes) to prevent an overexuberant blink response. Establish that the needle-syringe axis is in the iris plane and insert the needle tip just past the corneal endothelium, avoiding both the iris and anterior lens capsule.

8. Move the index finger against the syringe plunger to inject or aspirate up to 0.1 mL. (The entire anterior chamber volume is approximately 300 µL or 0.3 mL.)

9. Instill one additional drop of antibiotic.

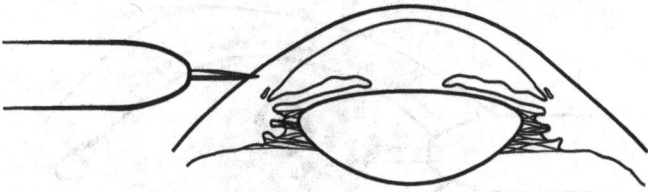

Figure 4-1a

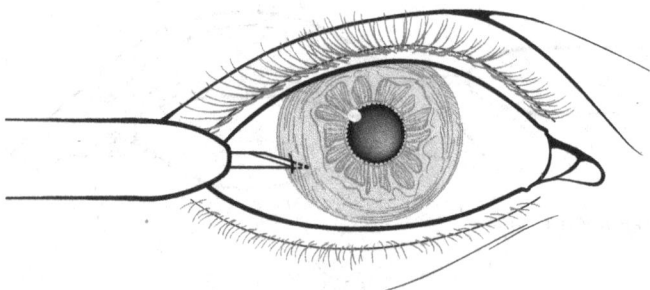

Figure 4-1b

5

Posterior Sub-Tenons Injection

INDICATIONS

Alternative method for anesthetizing the eye

EQUIPMENT

- Lid speculum
- 5-cc syringe
- Posterior sub-Tenons-cannula/or BSS cannula
- 2% lidocaine
- Westcott scissors
- 0.12 Cassie forceps
- Bipolar cautery

TECHNIQUE

1. Draw up 3 cc of lidocaine into the syringe and attach cannula.
2. Place lid speculum into eye.

3. In the inferonasal fornix, make a full-thickness conjunctival and sub-Tenons buttonhole incision using the Westcott scissors (Fig. 5-1).
4. Insert the closed scissor blades into the incision and spread to lyse adhesions along the globe.
5. Pass the cannula through the incision and posterior along the contour of the globe until the hub of the cannula is flush with the conjunctiva and perpendicular to the globe (Fig. 5-2).
6. Inject anesthetic slowly. There should be little or no resistance to the injection.
7. If desired, cauterize the incision closed.

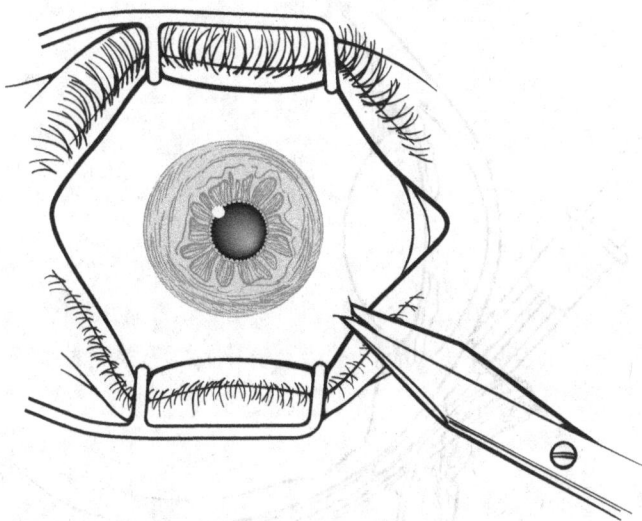

Figure 5-1

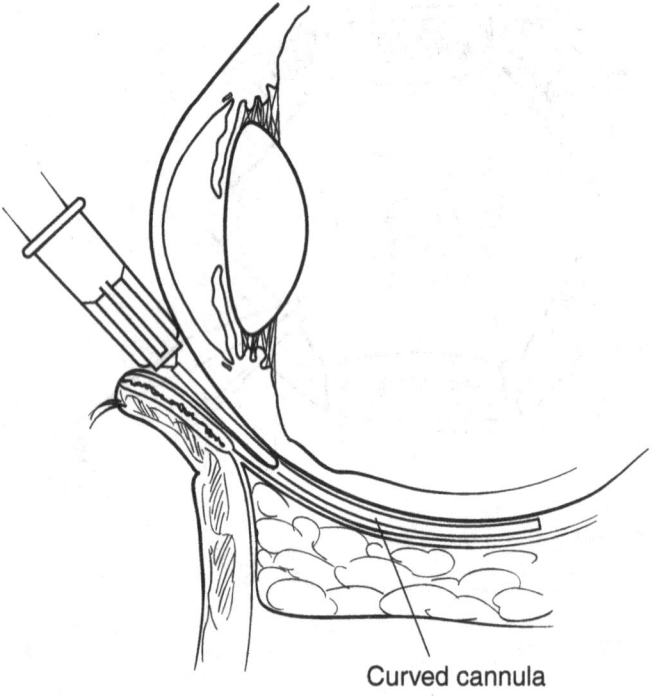

Curved cannula

Figure 5-2

6

Chalazion Excision

INDICATIONS

For incision and drainage of chalazia

EQUIPMENT

- Chalazion curette
- Chalazion clamp
- Bard-Parker #11 blade
- 3-cc Syringe
- Lidocaine 2% with epinephrine
- Topical proparacaine or tetracaine
- Topical antibiotic (eg, gentamicin)
- Povidone 5% solution
- 30-Gauge needle
- Sterile cotton tips
- Westcott scissors
- 0.3 Cassie forceps
- Sterile eye drape
- 2 Eye patches
- Tape
- Erythromycin ointment
- Ice pack

TECHNIQUE

1. Obtain informed surgical consent.
2. Place topical proparacaine into the eye.
3. Inject lidocaine with epinephrine with 30-gauge needle on 3-cc syringe to anesthetize eyelid.
4. Clean eyelid skin with 5% povidone solution.
5. Place 1 drop of topical antibiotic.
6. Drape the eye with sterile eye drape.
7. Place chalazion clamp across chalazion. Tighten clamp and evert eyelid. (Fig. 6-1).
8. Make a vertical incision perpendicular to the lid margin in the conjunctiva and tarsus across the center of the chalazion with #11 blade. Do not violate the lid margin (Fig. 6-2).
9. Use chalazion curette to lyse adhesions within chalazion.
10. Remove lipogranulomatous material using sterile cotton tips and curette. (Fig. 6-3).
11. Use forceps and Westcott scissors to remove cyst wall (optional) (Fig. 6-4).
12. Remove chalazion clamp.
13. Place erythromycin ointment into eye and pressure patch.
14. Place ice pack over dressing to reduce swelling.

NOTES

May use corneal shield to protect ocular surface.

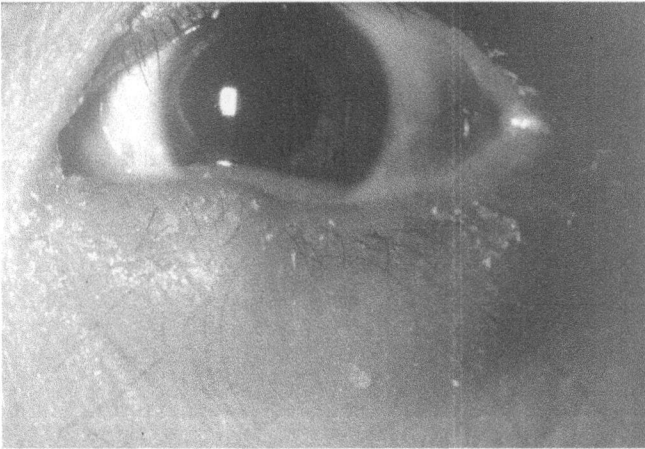

Figure 6-1

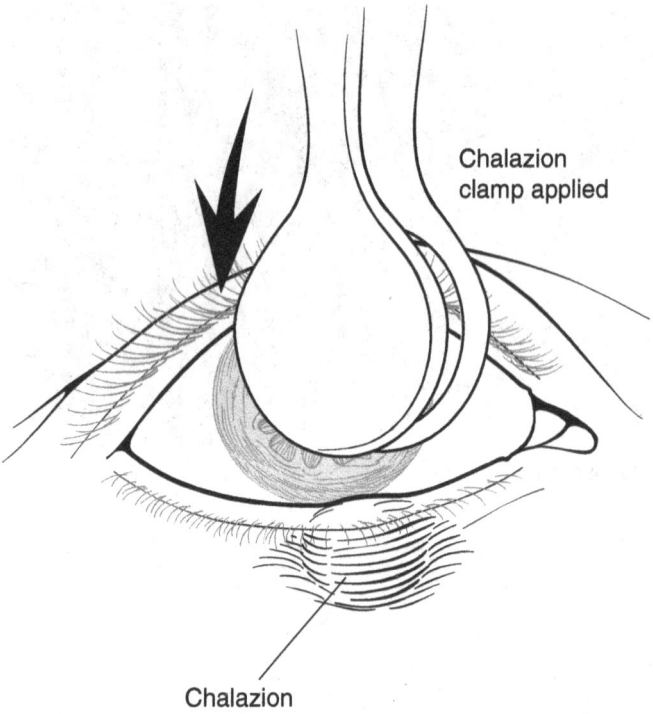

Chalazion
clamp applied

Chalazion

Figure 6-2

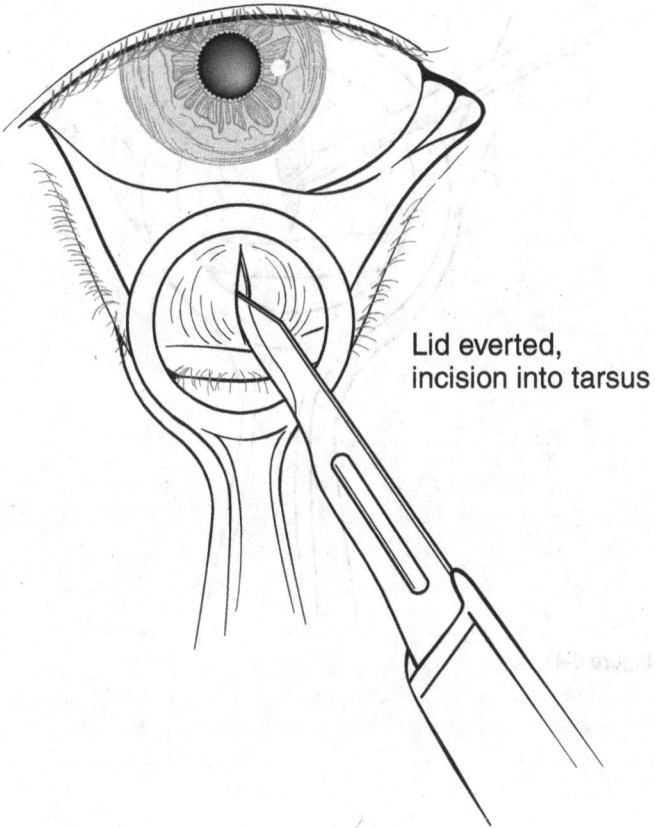

Lid everted,
incision into tarsus

Figure 6-3

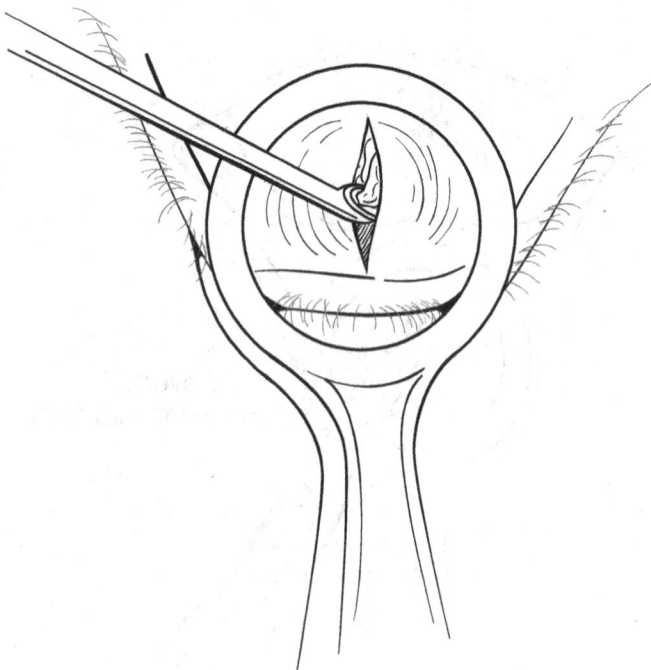

Figure 6-4

7

Conjunctival Biopsy

INDICATIONS

For obtaining tissue specimen for the diagnosis of sarcoidosis, ocular cicatricial pemphigoid, benign epithelial neoplasm, squamous cell carcinoma and dysplasias, primary acquired melanosis, nevi and melanoma, lymphoid disease

EQUIPMENT

- Broad-spectrum antibiotic drop
- Tetracaine eye drop
- Phenylephrine 2.5% eye drop
- 3-cc syringe
- 2% lidocaine
- 27- or 30-gauge needle
- Balanced salt solution (BSS) eye drop
- Wire-type eyelid speculum
- Sterile cotton-tipped applicators
- Sterile toothed forceps, 0.12 mm
- Sterile Westcott scissors, curved and blunt-tipped
- Disposable low-temperature thermal cautery
- Suture (type and gauge unimportant)

- Absorbent mount for specimen (filter paper)
- 10% formalin fixative solution in specimen container
- Ophthalmic erythromycin or bacitracin ointment

TECHNIQUE

1. Assemble the above supplies on a Mayo stand (or the equivalent) within arm's reach of the examination chair.
2. Place the patient in the examination chair and fully recline the chair.
4. Instill one drop each of antibiotic and tetracaine in the operative eye, instilling additional tetracaine as necessary during the procedure to achieve anesthesia.
5. Place the eyelid speculum (periodically instill BSS over the cornea during the remainder of the procedure to prevent corneal epithelial desiccation).
6. Direct the patient's gaze to optimally expose the planned biopsy site.
7. Soak a cotton-tipped applicator with tetracaine and phenylephrine and hold the medicated cotton tip against the planned biopsy site for 30 to 40 seconds. Alternatively, lidocaine can be injected under the conjunctiva to balloon up the biopsy site (Fig. 7-1).
8. Grasp one border of the planned biopsy site with toothed forceps and incise the conjunctiva with Westcott scissors. Next, undermine the biopsy area with the scissors, separating conjunctiva from the underlying Tenon's capsule and incise along the conjunctival borders (Figs. 7-2, 7-3, and 7-4).
9. Achieve hemostasis by gentle pressure with cotton-tipped applicator or with low-temperature cautery of vessels if necessary.
10. Remove the eyelid speculum and place ophthalmic ointment in the lower fornix of the operative eye.
11. Tag a margin of the conjunctival specimen with a suture and indicate which margin is tagged on the pathology requisition form (eg, nasal margin sutured).

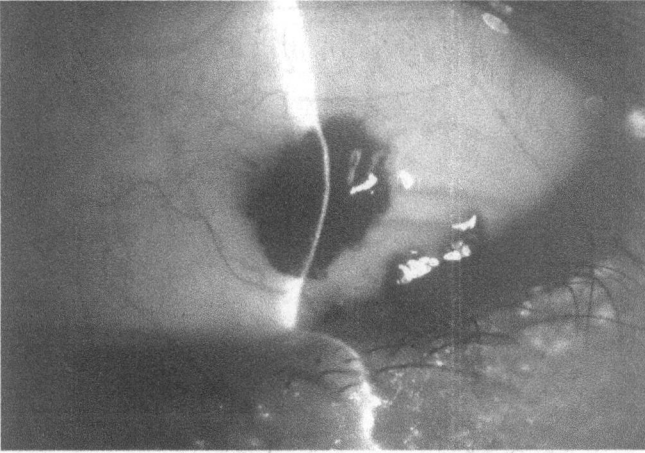

Figure 7-1

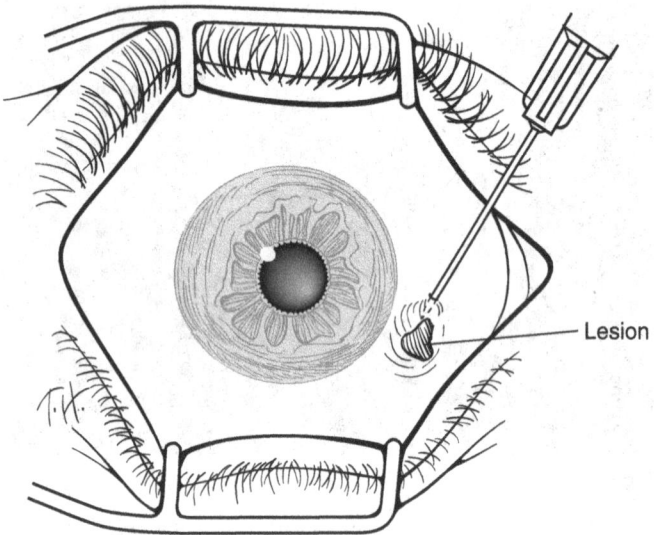

Figure 7-2

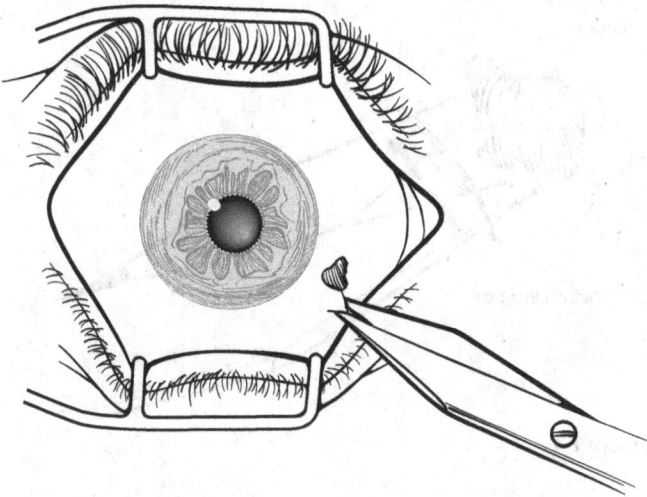

Figure 7-3

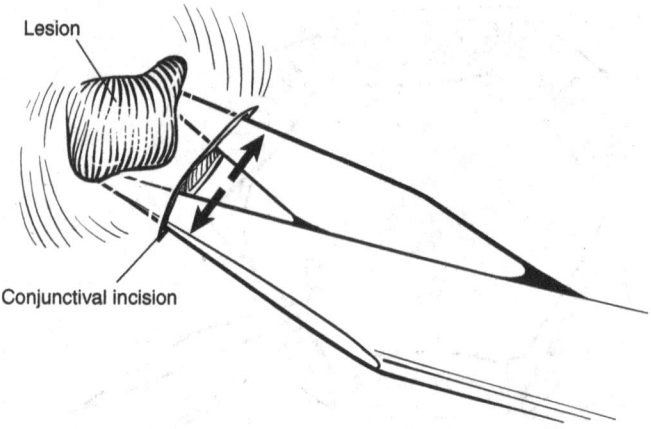

Figure 7-4

Place the specimen on an absorbent mount such as filter paper and allow to dry 15 to 20 seconds. Place the specimen in the specimen container with fixative and send to the pathology lab.

CAUTIONS

Avoid painting the margins of a conjunctival biopsy with a methylene blue or toluidine blue marking pen as these aqueous based dyes will "bleed" into the tissue. Dyed tissue is difficult for the pathologist to evaluate.

Conjunctival epithelial defects can be extremely painful, occasionally requiring narcotic analgesics such as Vicodin or Percocet.

8

Corneal Biopsy

INDICATIONS

Diagnosis of corneal ulcer unresponsive to medication and culture negative (ie, those ulcers associated with mycobacteria, fungus, *Acanthamoeba*, and *Streptococcus*, among others)

EQUIPMENT

- Broad-spectrum antibiotic drops
- Tetracaine eye drops
- Wire-type eyelid speculum
- Corneal trephine, 2-3 mm dermatologic type
- Toothed forceps, 0.12 mm
- Crescent blade on handle
- 15-degree supersharp blade
- Pathology specimen container

TECHNIQUE

1. Assemble the above supplies on a Mayo stand (or the equivalent).
2. Position patient supine under operating microscope, instill one drop each of antibiotic and tetracaine in the

operative eye, instilling additional tetracaine as necessary during the procedure to achieve anesthesia.

3. Place the eyelid speculum and instruct the patient to remain still. If necessary enlist an assistant to help immobilize the patient's head.

4. Direct the patient's gaze to optimally expose the planned biopsy site.

5. Place corneal trephine against the cornea straddling both healthy and diseased portions if possible. Gently roll the trephine between the thumb and index finger and create a partial-thickness wound. (Fig. 8-1a and 8-1b).

6. Lift an edge of the trephined cornea with 0.12 forceps and dissect this partial-thickness biopsy away from the rest of the cornea with a crescent blade (Figs. 8-2a, 8-2b, and 8-3).

7. Remove the eyelid speculum, instill an additional antibiotic drop, and send the patient home advising him or her to continue using the antimicrobial regimen used previously until otherwise directed.

8. Place the specimen in the specimen container and transport directly to pathology lab for further microbiologic and histologic evaluation.

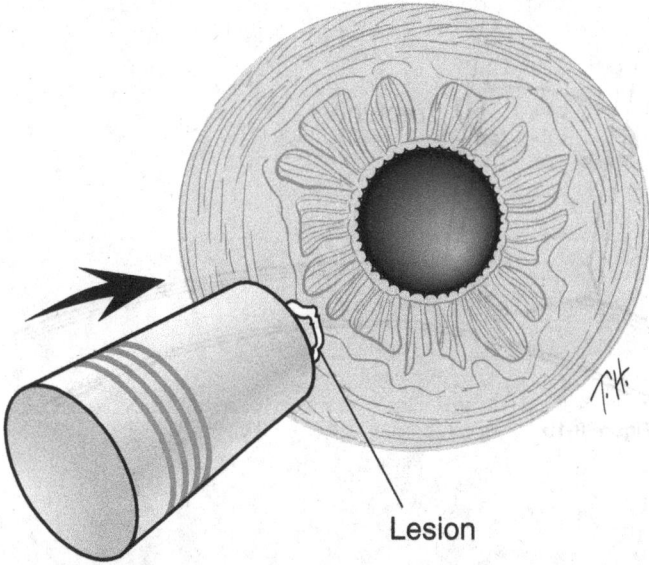

Lesion

Figure 8-1a

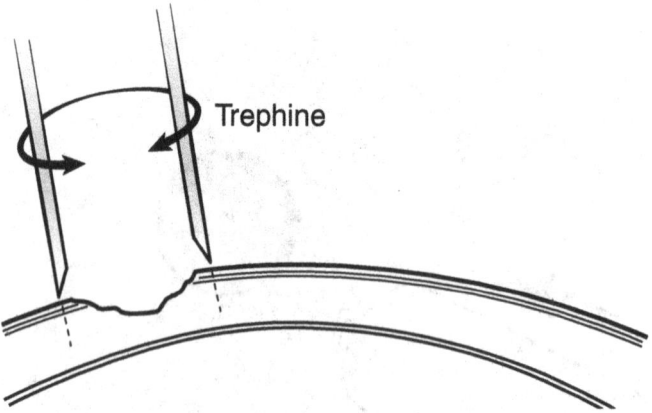

Figure 8-1b

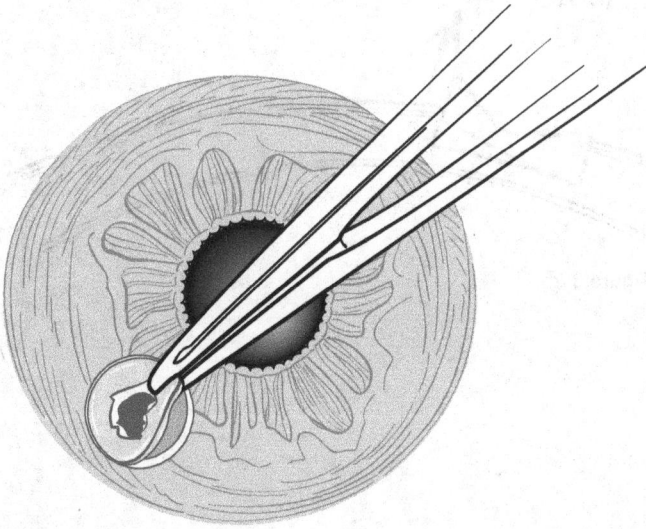

Figure 8-2a

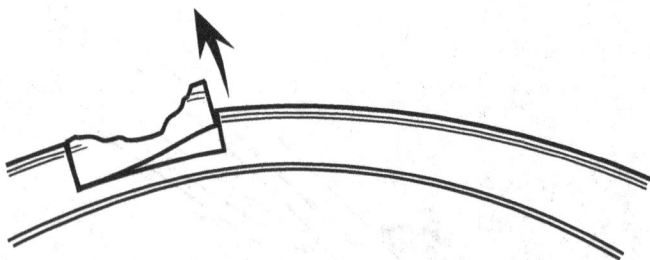

Figure 8-2b

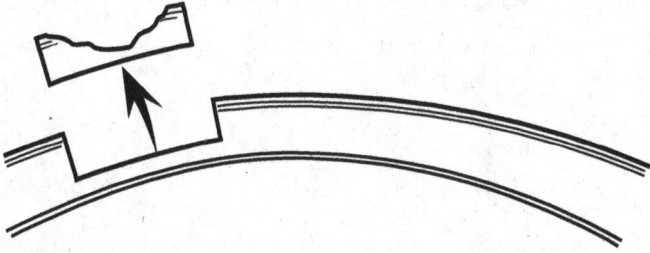

Figure 8-3

9

Corneal Glue Placement

INDICATIONS

Corneal perforations or ulcerations smaller than 1.5 mm in diameter as a temporizing measure until penetrating keratoplasty can be performed. (Contraindications include iris or vitreous prolapse and corneal perforations larger than 1.5 mm.)

EQUIPMENT

- Broad-spectrum antibiotic
- Proparacaine eye drop
- Wire-type eyelid speculum
- Medical-grade cyanoacrylate adhesive with plastic storage well
- Sterile cellulose sponge spears
- 30-gauge hypodermic needle
- 1-cc syringe
- Fluorescein strip
- Bandage contact lens

TECHNIQUE

1. Assemble the above supplies on a Mayo stand (or the equivalent) within arm's reach of the examination chair.
2. Place the patient in the examination chair and fully recline the chair.
3. Don magnifying loupes.
4. Instill one drop each of antibiotic and proparacaine in the operative eye.
5. Load 0.2 cc of cyanoacrylate adhesive from a plastic storage well into a 1-cc syringe and attach a 30-gauge needle to the syringe.
6. Place the eyelid speculum.
7. Direct the patient's gaze to optimally expose the corneal perforation.
8. Debride and dry the corneal defect and corneal surface immediately surrounding the defect with cellulose spears (Fig. 9-1a and 9-1b).
9. Drop one to two drops of adhesive onto the dried corneal defect and a small part of the surrounding cornea (Fig. 9-2).
10. The adhesive will polymerize immediately on contact with the eye. Wait for 1 minute to permit full polymerization.
11. Bring the patient to the seated position in the examination chair and paint the cornea with a moistened fluorescein strip. If the defect has not been completely sealed by the adhesive, as evidenced by a positive Seidel test, repeat steps 7, 8 and 9.
12. Remove the eyelid speculum and place a bandage contact lens over the cornea to protect the palpebral conjunctiva from the rough surface of the dried adhesive (Fig. 9-3).
13. Instill an additional drop of antibiotic and discharge the patient.

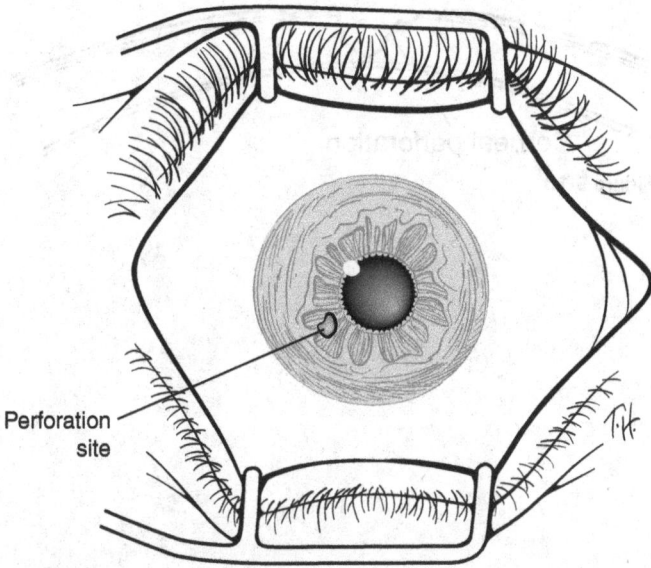

Perforation site

Figure 9-1a

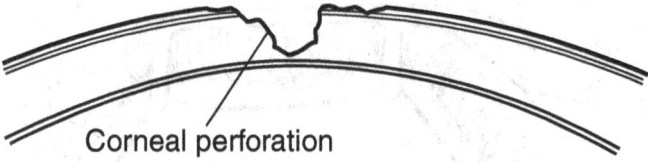

Figure 9-1b

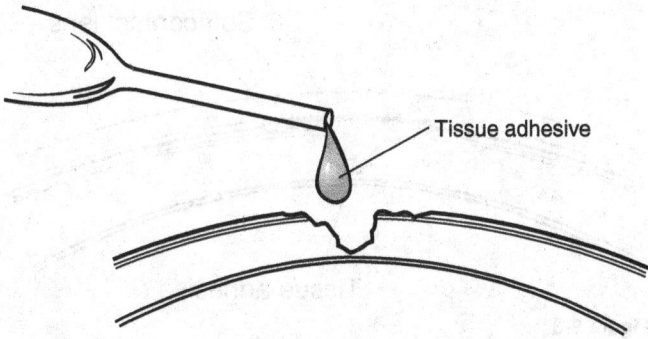

Tissue adhesive

Figure 9-2

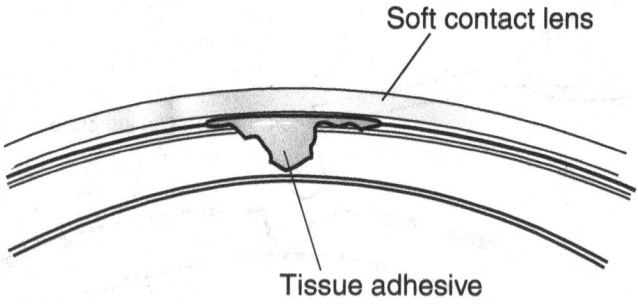

Soft contact lens

Tissue adhesive

Figure 9-3

CAUTIONS

In time corneal epithelial cells will undermine the cyanoacrylate adhesive applied to surface defects of the cornea and cause the adhesive to eventually slough off of the cornea. Adhesive application therefore should be viewed as a temporary solution to corneal perforations.

Part 2

Glaucoma

Discussion

10

Bleb Needling

INDICATIONS

Poorly functioning glaucoma bleb due to fibrosis of the trabeculectomy flap or loculation within the bleb (Fig. 10-1)

EQUIPMENT

- Wire lid speculum
- 25-gauge needle
- 1-cc tuberculin syringe
- Antibiotic drop
- Cotton swab
- Fluorescein strip

TECHNIQUE

1. Insert lid speculum.
2. Place a drop of proparacaine into the eye. Moistening a cotton swab with proparacaine and holding this on the conjunctival surface lateral to the filtering bleb can give additional, deeper local anesthesia.
3. Place a drop of an antibiotic into the eye.

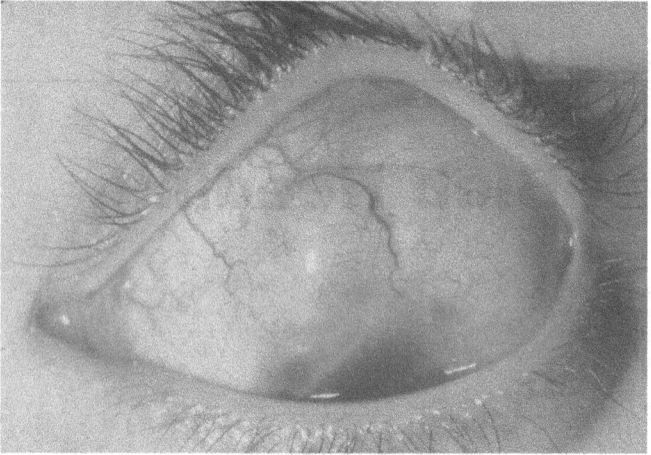

Figure 10-1

4. Starting several millimeters lateral to the bleb, insert the needle bevel up under the conjunctiva and tunnel towards the bleb (Fig. 10-2).
5. Under direct visualization, lyse fibrosis within the bleb.
6. Withdraw the needle.
7. Check the entry site with the fluorescein strip for leakage of aqueous.

NOTES

If successful, the bleb will fill with fluid and the intraocular pressure will fall.

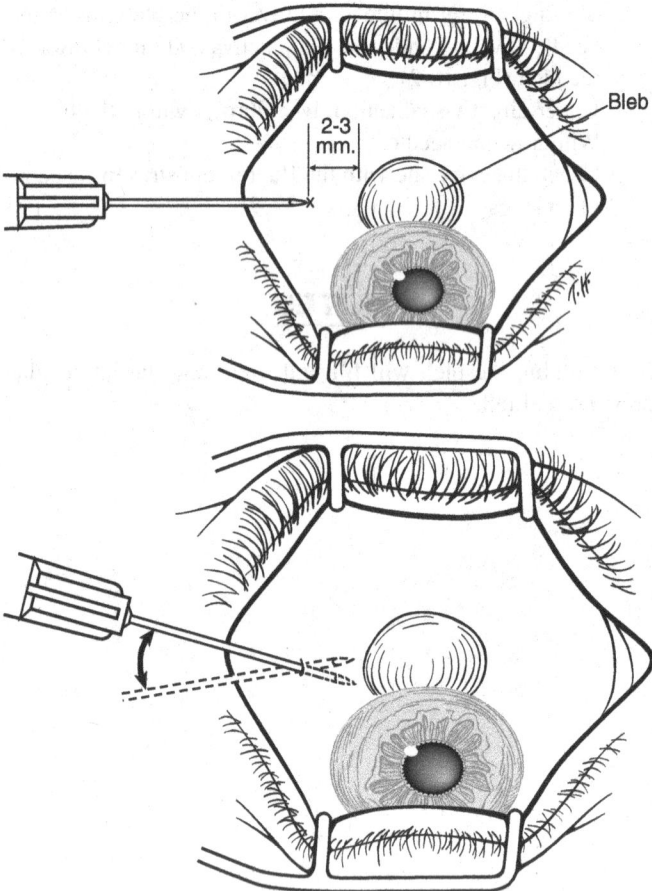

2-3 mm.

Bleb

Figure 10-2

11

Subconjunctival 5-Fluorouracil Injection

INDICATIONS

Subconjunctival 5-fluorouracil injections are used to reduce post-trabeculectomy fibrosis to preserve and protect the filtration function of the bleb.

EQUIPMENT

- Broad-spectrum antibiotic
- Proparacaine
- 0.1 cc of 50 mg/mL 5-fluorouracil (5-FU)
- 1-cc tuberculin syringe
- 25-gauge needle
- Chemotherapeutic disposal bin
- Smooth Bishop Harmon forceps

TECHNIQUE

1. Place a drop of proparacaine into the eye. Moistening a cotton swab with proparacaine and holding this on the conjunctival surface can give additional, deeper local anesthesia.
2. Place a drop of antibiotic into the eye.
3. Draw up 0.1 cc of 50 mg/mL 5-FU into a 1-cc tuberculin syringe with a 25-gauge needle.
4. Tent up the conjunctiva 180 degrees from the filtering site with a smooth forceps.
5. Insert the needle beneath the conjunctiva and inject 0.1 cc of 5-FU (Fig. 11-1).
6. Discard the needle and syringe in a chemotherapeutic-approved disposal bin.
7. This procedure can generally be repeated three times to reduce post-trabeculectomy bleb fibrosis.
8. We recommend that if injecting closer to the trabeculectomy site than indicated above, that this be done in consultation with a glaucoma specialist.

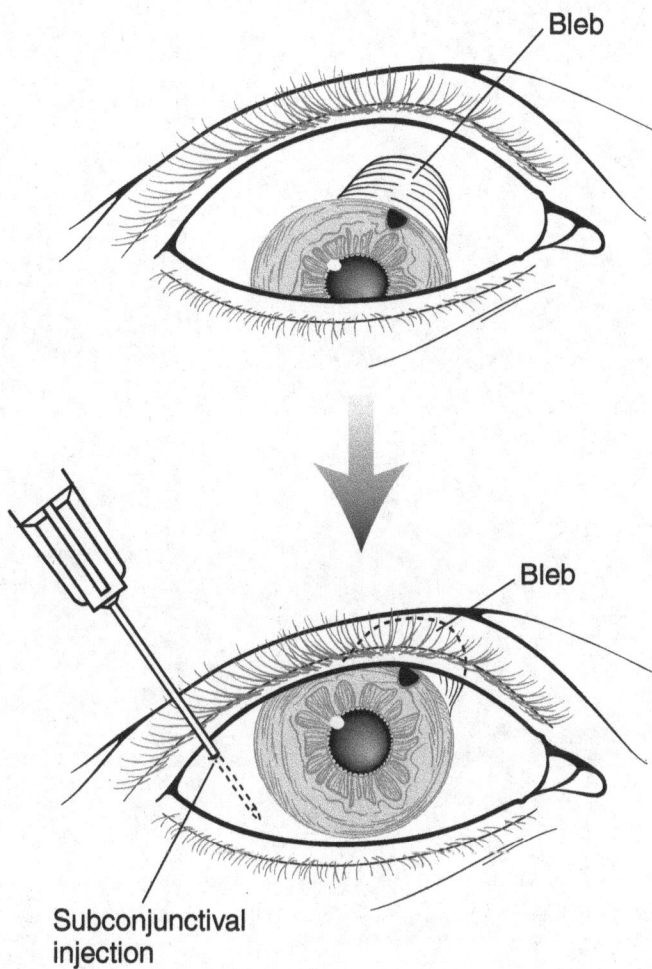

Figure 11-1

12

Laser Suture Lysis

INDICATIONS

Laser suture lysis can be used to cut subconjunctival sutures in patients who have undergone extracapsular cataract extraction or trabeculectomy with a scleral flap sutures.

EQUIPMENT

- Laser suture lysis lens
- Proparacaine
- Argon slit lamp laser
- Fluorescein strip

TECHNIQUE

1. Place a drop of proparacaine into the eye.
2. Laser settings:
   - 50-micron spot size
   - Argon green wavelength
   - 700 to 900 mW power
   - 0.1-second duration
   - 10 to 25x slit lamp magnification

3. Have the patient focus on a fixation target with the other eye to reduce ocular movement.
4. Place the laser suture lysis lens across the stitch to be cut (Fig. 12-1).
5. Focus the laser beam on the stitch over the sclera.
6. Narrow the focus beam to its sharpest and deliver a laser pulse (Figs. 12-2 and 12-3).
7. Begin at the lowest power setting and deliver several pulses per stitch before increasing the laser power.
8. With lysis of sutures in extracapsular cataract extraction and trabeculectomy flap release, the wound should be assessed by the Seidel method after completion of laser suture lysis.
9. With lysis of trabeculectomy scleral flap sutures, digital pressure should be applied to the posterior lip of the flap if increased aqueous shunting is desired, the bleb should be checked by the Seidel method, and the intraocular pressure should also be assessed.

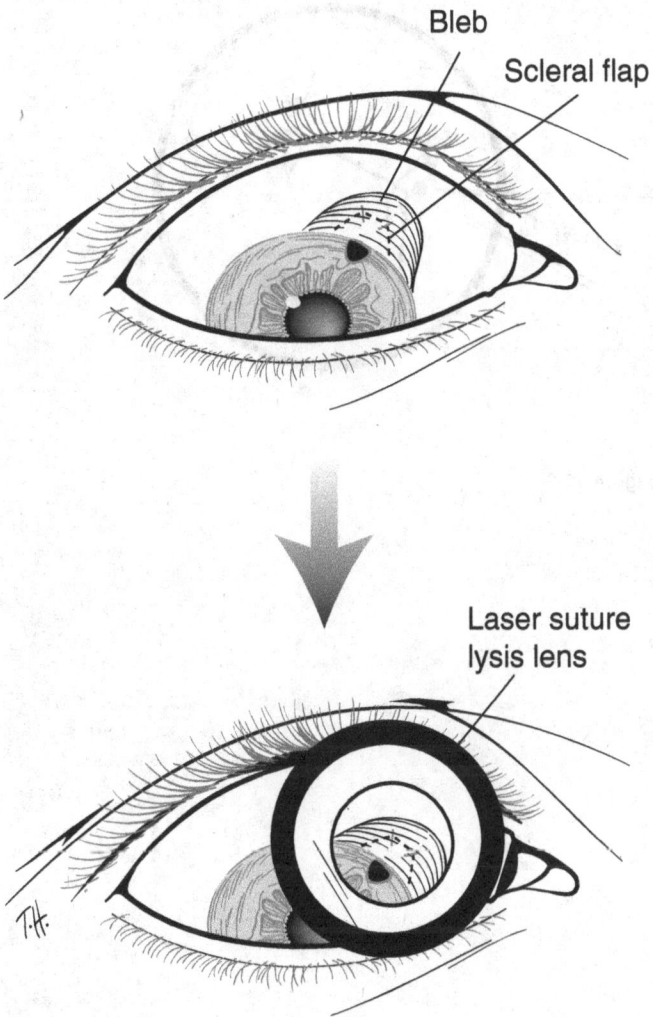

Figure 12-1

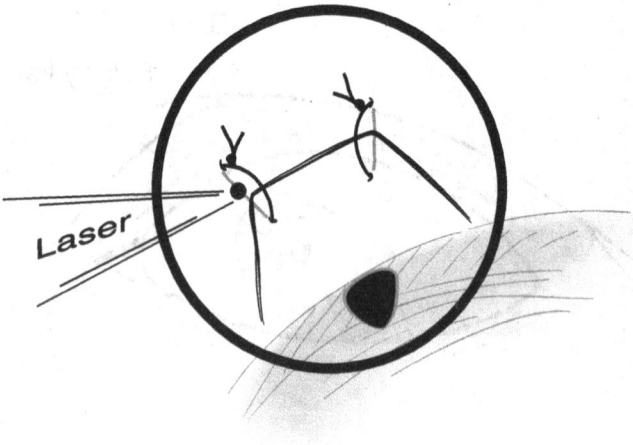

Figure 12-2

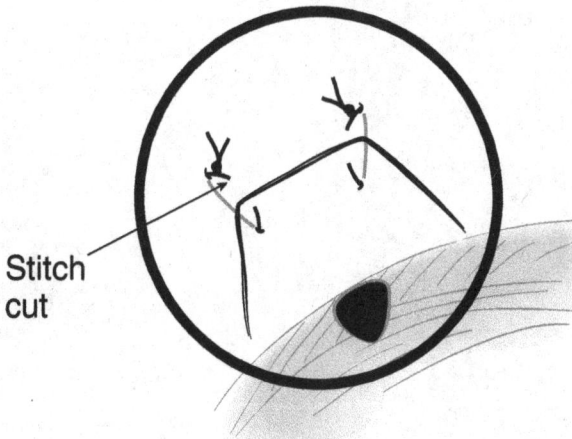

Stitch
cut

Figure 12-3

13

Autologous Blood Patching for Overfiltering Blebs

INDICATIONS

For use in decreasing the aqueous outflow following glaucoma filtration surgery.

EQUIPMENT

- 25-gauge straight needle
- 1- to 3-cc syringe
- Alcohol wipe
- Topical proparacaine
- Smooth Bishop Harmon forceps
- Topical antibiotic of choice
- 4 × 4 Cotton gauze
- Tourniquet

TECHNIQUE

1. Place a drop of proparacaine into the eye.
2. Place a drop of antibiotic into the eye.
3. Draw 1 cc of blood from a peripheral vein.
4. Tent up the conjunctiva with smooth Bishop Harmon forceps either nasal or temporal to the bleb. Insert the needle (bevel up) 2 to 3 mm from the elevated bleb to reduce the chance of conjunctival puncture in the bleb region (Fig. 13-1).
5. Tunnel beneath the conjunctiva until the tip of the needle is in the bleb-enclosed subconjunctival space.
6. Inject about 0.1 cc of the patient's blood into the bleb and remove the needle.
7. Have the patient lay flat for about 10 minutes while the blood clots to reduce the chance of a iatrogenic hyphema.
8. Perform a Seidel test to assess for a bleb leak.
9. Wait 1 hour and recheck the intraocular pressure.
10. Repeat steps 3 through 9 if necessary.

Blood beneath bleb

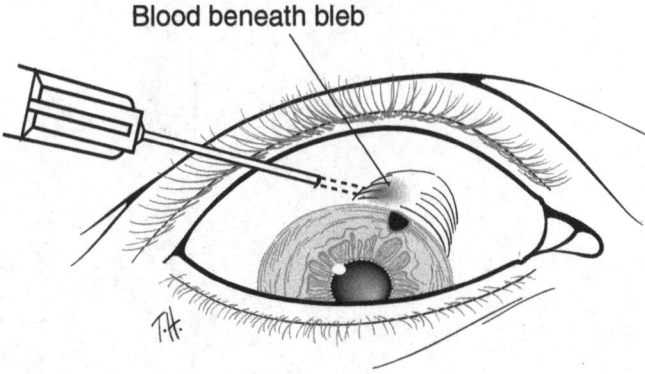

Figure 13-1

14

Laser Gonioplasty

INDICATIONS

Plateau iris

EQUIPMENT

- Argon laser
- Apraclonidine 1% drops
- Pilocarpine 1% drops

TECHNIQUE

1. Place a drop of apraclonidine and pilocarpine 1% in the eye 1 hour prior to the procedure.
2. Laser settings:
   - Argon green wavelength
   - 200 to 500 μm spot size
   - 0.1- to 0.5-second duration
   - 200 to 500 mW power
3. Aim the laser at the far peripheral iris. The procedure may be performed with or without a contact lens. The desired result is a visible contraction of iris tissue. Place 4 to 6

spots per quadrant over the entire circumference of the iris (Fig. 14-1).

4. Postoperatively, place a drop of apraclonidine in the eye. Check for acute intraocular pressure spike 1 hour after the procedure. Inflammation can be controlled with a short course of prednisolone acetate 1% (1 drop qid for 5 days).

PITFALLS

Complications of gonioplasty include acute IOP spike and iritis. The diagnosis of plateau iris requires the presence of a patent peripheral iridectomy.

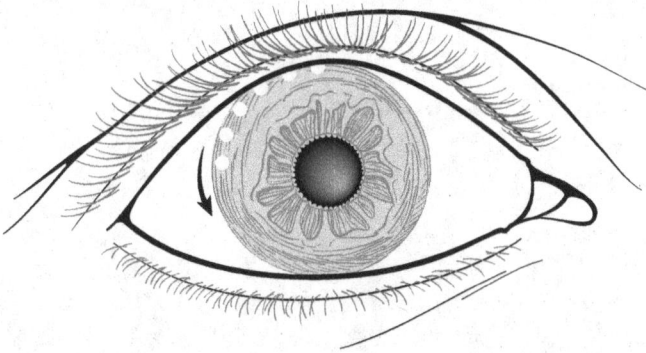

Figure 14-1

15

Laser Peripheral Iridotomy

INDICATIONS

Angle closure glaucoma secondary to pupillary block.

Prevention of angle closure glaucoma in eyes at risk for developing pupillary block.

EQUIPMENT

- Condensing contact lens (ie, Abraham)
- Coupling solution
- Topical anesthetic (proparacaine)
- Pilocarpine 1%
- Apraclonidine 1%

TECHNIQUE

1. Place a drop of pilocarpine and apraclonidine in the eye one half hour prior to treatment.
2. Place a drop of proparacaine in the eye.
3. Place the condensing contact lens on the eye with coupling solution.

4. The ideal iridotomy site should be peripheral and covered by the upper eyelid (Fig. 15-1). The 12:00 position should be avoided because bubbles may interfere with completion of the iridotomy. An iris crypt is easier to penetrate.

5. Argon laser settings
   - 50-μm spot size
   - 0.02- to 0.1-second duration
   - 600 to 1000 mW power
   Nd:Yag laser settings
   - 2 to 6 mJ energy

6. The Nd:Yag laser works well for most eyes. The argon laser is more difficult with lighter irides. In darker irides the argon laser can be used to coagulate and thin the stroma and decrease incidence of hemorrhage. The Nd:Yag laser can then be used to make a hole through the pigment epithelium, often with a single shot (Fig. 15-2).

7. Bleeding may occur from the iridotomy site. This can be controlled with compression of the eye using the contact lens.

8. Postoperatively, place a drop of apraclonidine in the eye. Check for acute intraocular pressure spike 1 hour after the procedure. Inflammation can be controlled with a short course of prednisolone acetate 1% (1 drop qid for 5 days).

PITFALLS

The cornea may be cloudy in acute angle closure. In this case, decrease the IOP medically and perform the LPI once the cornea clears. Topical glycerin drops can be useful to clear the epithelial edema. Potential complications of LPI include bleeding, IOP spike, lens damage, and retinal detachment.

NOTES

When the iris is penetrated, there is frequently a gush of pigment and fluid through the iridotomy site. Transillumination of the iris is useful to confirm the patency of the iridotomy.

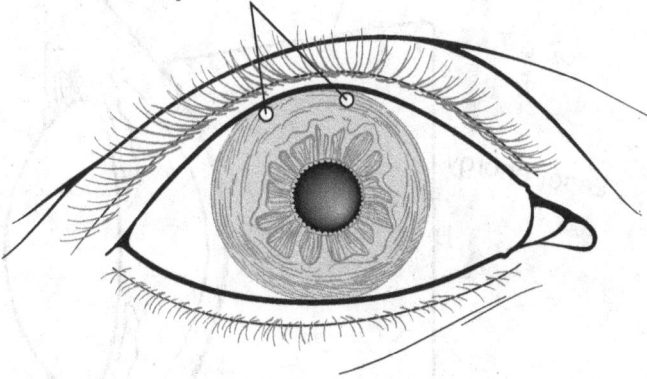

Ideal peripheral
iridectomy sites

Figure 15-1

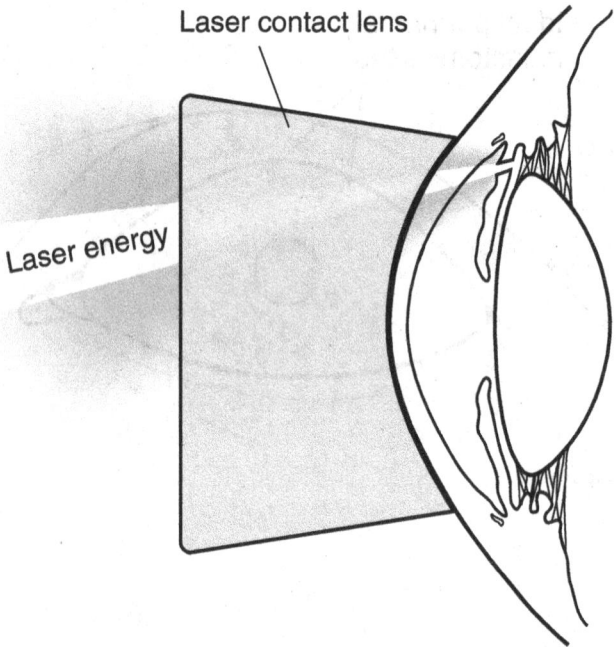

Figure 15-2

16

Argon Laser Trabeculoplasty

INDICATIONS

Primary open-angle glaucoma
Pigmentary glaucoma
Pseudoexfoliation glaucoma

EQUIPMENT

- Argon laser
- Contact goniolens
- Coupling solution (goniosol)
- Topical anesthetic (proparacaine)
- Apraclonidine

TECHNIQUE

1. Pretreat the eye with 1 drop of apraclonidine 1 hour prior to the procedure.
2. Place a drop of proparacaine in the eye.

3. Place the contact goniolens on the eye using coupling solution (Fig. 16-1).
4. Initial argon laser settings
   - Argon green wavelength
   - 50 μm spot size
   - 0.1-second duration
   - 300 to 1000 mW power
5. Aim for the junction of the anterior nonpigmented and posterior pigmented trabecular meshwork (Fig. 16-2). Titrate the power to the minimum needed to achieve the desired result of a blanching of the trabecular meshwork or the production of a small bubble.
6. Place 40 to 50 spots over 180 degrees of the angle with two beam-widths between spots.
7. Postoperatively, place a drop of apraclonidine in the eye. Check for acute intraocular pressure spike 1 hour after the procedure. Inflammation can be controlled with a short course of prednisolone acetate 1% (1 drop qid for 5 days).

PITFALLS

Complications of ALT include acute IOP spike, iritis, and rarely the formation of peripheral anterior synechiae.

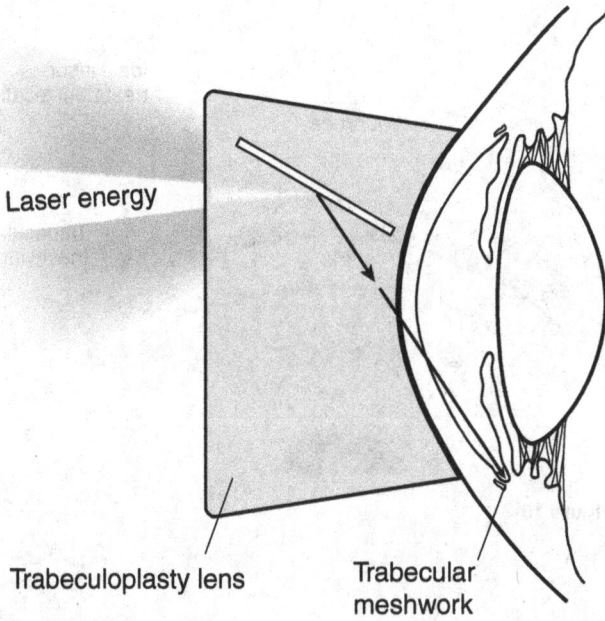

Laser energy

Trabeculoplasty lens

Trabecular
meshwork

Figure 16-1

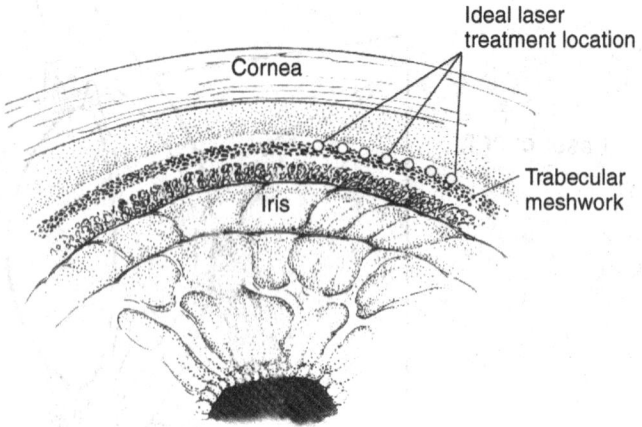

Figure 16-2

Part 3

Cataract

17

Nd:Yag Laser Posterior Capsulotomy

INDICATIONS

For removal of posterior capsule opacifications or fibrosis obstructing visual axis following cataract surgery

EQUIPMENT

- Topical anesthetic (proparacaine or tetracaine drops)
- Dilating drops
- Pressure-lowering drops (eg, Apraclonidine 0.5%, Brimonidine 0.2%, Timolol 0.5%)
- Nd:Yag laser
- Contact lens (ie, Abraham-Yag lens, Peyman lens)
- Methylcellulose (Goniosol)
- Apraclonidine 1% drops

TECHNIQUE

1. Assemble the necessary instruments and supplies.
2. Dilate the patient 30 minutes prior to the procedure.
3. Anesthetize the eye with several drops of topical anesthetic (proparacaine drops). Premedicate the patient with pressure-lowering drops.
4. Position the patient comfortably at the Nd:Yag laser.
5. Put Goniosol on the lens (avoid air bubbles!), have the patient look up, and insert the lens into the eye.
6. Superimpose the two red laser focusing beams on the posterior capsule. To avoid pitting the lens, aim the focusing beam slightly posterior to the posterior capsule (Fig. 17-1).
7. Use a lower power setting of approximately 1.0 mJ. This setting can slowly be increased by 0.2-mJ increments to reach effective cutting power.
8. One can cut the capsule in a circular pattern or a cruciate pattern. The circular pattern reduces the possibility of lens pits in the visual axis (Fig. 17-2).
9. Post-laser treatment give one drop of pressure-lowering drops.
10. Measure intraocular pressure 1 hour post-laser treatment to check for pressure spike.
11. Treat patient with 3 to 5 days of topical steroids.

NOTES

Yag:Nd laser treatment of the posterior capsule carries a risk of localized corneal epithelial damage, marking or dislocating the lens, and retinal detachment. For diabetic patients, try to make the capsulotomy as large as possible. Lens pits from laser disruption of the lens surface usually does not affect vision and is not noticed by the patient.

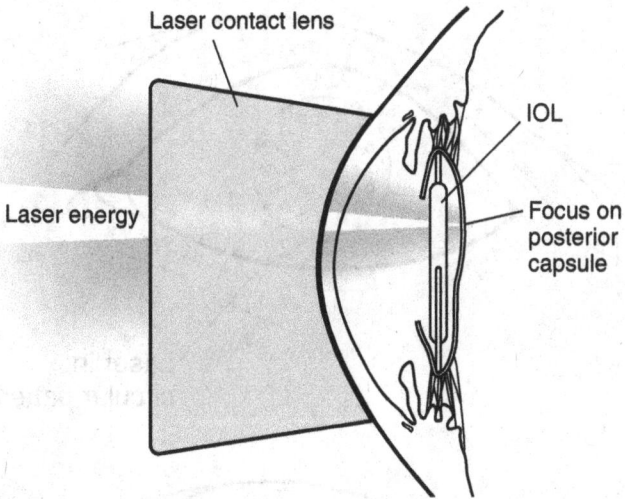

Figure 17-1

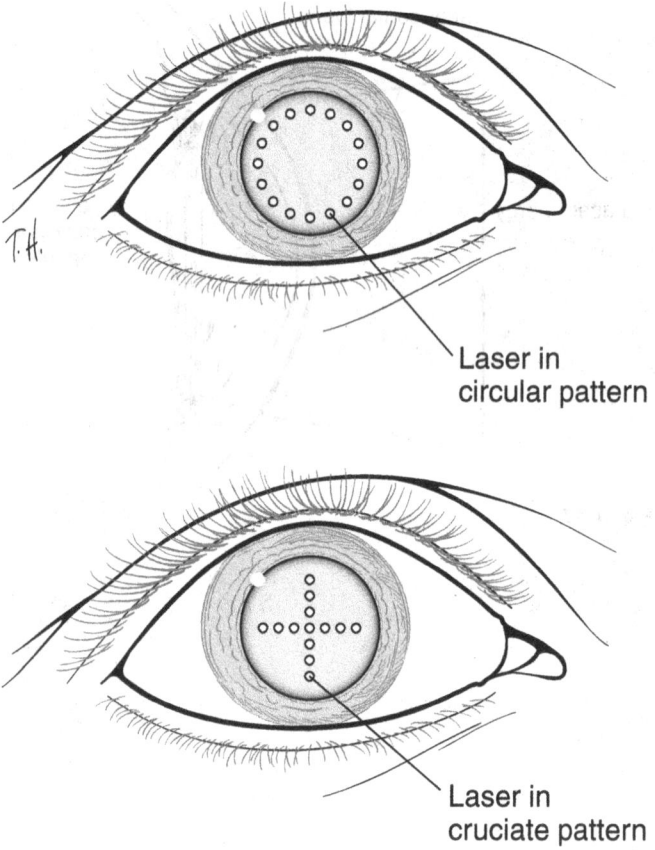

Laser in
circular pattern

Laser in
cruciate pattern

Figure 17-2

18

Nd:Yag Laser Vitreolysis

INDICATIONS

For severing of a vitreous strand attached to a corneal incision following cataract surgery to prevent or treat cystoid macular edema.

EQUIPMENT

- Topical anesthetic (proparacaine or tetracaine drops)
- Pilocarpine 1% or 2%
- Pressure-lowering drop (ie, Iopidine 0.5%, Alphagan, Timoptic 0.5%)
- Nd:Yag laser
- Contact lens (ie, Abraham-Yag lens, Peyman lens)
- Methylcellulose solution (Goniosol)
- Apraclonidine drops

TECHNIQUE

1. Assemble the necessary instruments and supplies.
2. Anesthetize the eye with several drops of topical anesthetic (proparacaine drops). Premedicate the patient with the pressure-lowering drops.

3. Place a drop of pilocarpine into the eye to constrict the pupil and place the vitreous strand under a little tension.
4. Position the patient comfortably at the Nd:Yag laser machine.
5. Put Goniosol on the lens (avoid air bubbles!), have the patient look up, and insert the lens into the eye.
6. Aim the laser focusing beam on the vitreous strand in the anterior chamber. Try to find a portion of the strand away from the cornea (Fig. 18-1).
7. Use a lower power setting of approximately 1.0 mJ. This setting can slowly be increased by 0.2-mJ increments to reach effective cutting power.
8. After laser treatment give one drop of pressure-lowering medication.
9. Measure intraocular pressure 1 hour post-laser treatment to check for pressure spike.
10. Treat patient with 3 to 5 days of topical steroids.

NOTES

Yag:Nd laser vitreolysis is more successful for small single strands of vitreous in the anterior chamber. For larger strands that distort the pupil, one should consider anterior vitrectomy.

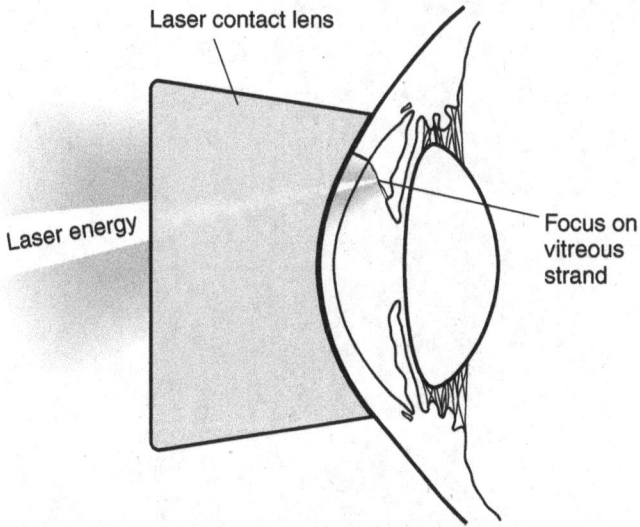

Figure 18-1

Part 4

Neuro-ophthalmology

19

Pharmacologic Testing of Abnormal Pupils

INDICATIONS

Anisocoria

EQUIPMENT

- Cocaine 4% to 10% drops
- Hydroxyamphetamine 1% drops
- Pilocarpine 0.125% drops

TECHNIQUE

1. Assemble the necessary supplies. The flow chart in Fig. 19-1 outlines the different drops and the testing pathways.
2. Suspicion of Horner's syndrome (miosis, ptosis, anisocoria pupillary size difference greater in dark than light) can be confirmed by instillation of topical cocaine 4% to 10% drops. A Horner's syndrome pupil does not dilate.

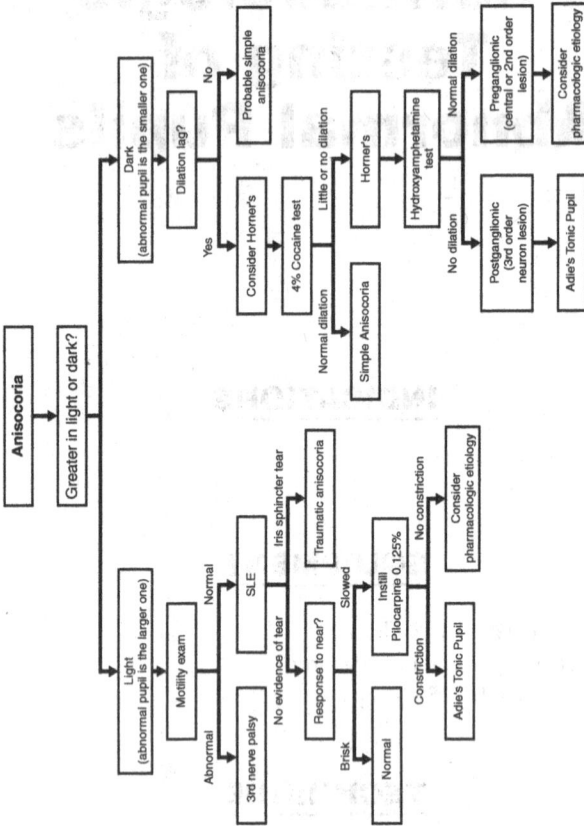

Figure 19-1

3. Preganglionic and postganglionic Horner's syndromes are differentiated by testing with 1% hydroxyamphetamine. If the pupil does not dilate, the postganglionic neuron is not intact.
4. Suspected Adie's tonic pupil can be confirmed with instillation of 0.125% pilocarpine in the dilated pupil. If the pupil constricts, the test is positive.

PITFALLS

Testing of pupils with pharmacologic agents should not be done within 24 hours of any eye drop use.

20

Tensilon Test

INDICATIONS

Tensilon testing is indicated for patients suspected of having intermittent diplopia or ptosis secondary to myasthenia gravis.

EQUIPMENT

- Tensilon (edrophonium) 10 mg/mL, 1-mL aliquot
- Atropine 0.4 mg
- Butterfly needle (25-gauge)
- Multiswitch stopcock
- Two 1-cc syringes
- One 10-cc syringe
- Normal saline
- Prism bars or loose prisms
- Ruler
- Camera (optional)
- Electrocardiograph

TECHNIQUE FOR PTOSIS EVALUATION

1. Draw up 1 cc of Tensilon (edrophonium) in the 1-cc syringe.
2. Draw up 5 to 6 cc of saline in the 10-cc syringe.
3. Draw up 0.4 mg of atropine in 1-cc syringe.
4. Insert butterfly needle into vein.
5. Measure vertical palpebral fissure height and superior margin reflex distance (MRD_1) prior to Tensilon administration and record measurements. Optional: Photograph lid position before injection (Fig. 20-1a).
6. Optional: Administer 0.4 mg of atropine IV and flush tubing with 1 cc saline. We premedicate all our patients with atropine.
7. Administer 0.2 cc of Tensilon and flush with 1 cc of saline.
8. Wait 1 minute and remeasure ptosis. Record and/or photograph.
9. If improvement, Tensilon test is positive and testing is concluded (Fig. 20-1b).
10. If no improvement occurs by 2 minutes, administer 0.4 cc of Tensilon and flush with 1 cc of saline.
11. Wait 1 minute and remeasure ptosis.
12. If no improvement, administer remainder of Tensilon (0.4 cc).
13. If still no improvement, Tensilon test is negative.

TECHNIQUE FOR DIPLOPIA EVALUATION

1. Draw up 1 cc of Tensilon in 1-cc syringe.
2. Draw up 5 to 6 cc of saline in 10-cc syringe.
3. Draw up 0.4 mg of atropine in 1-cc syringe.
4. Insert butterfly needle into vein.

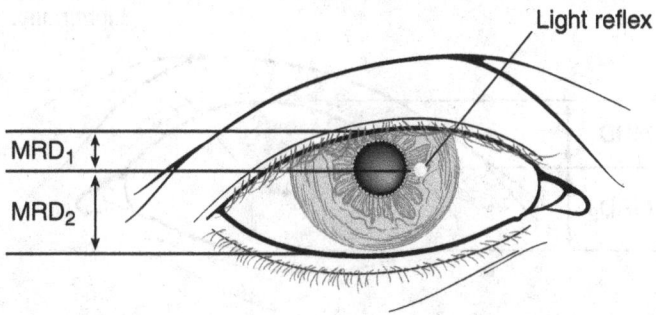

Figure 20-1a

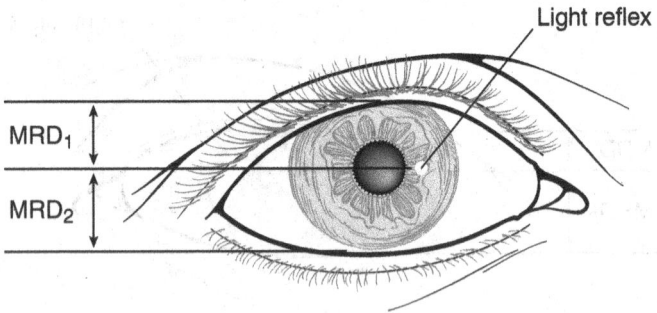

Figure 20-1b

5. Measure distance deviation with prism bars and record. Optional: Photograph both eyes to document misalignment.

6. Optional: Administer 0.4 mg of atropine IV and flush tubing with 1 cc saline. We premedicate all our patients with atropine.

7. Administer 0.2 to 0.3 cc of Tensilon and flush with 1 cc of saline.

8. Wait 1 minute and remeasure deviation. Record and/or photograph.

9. If improvement, Tensilon test is positive and testing is concluded.

10. If no improvement occurs by 2 minutes, administer 0.3 to 0.4 cc of Tensilon and flush with 1 cc of saline.

11. Wait 1 minute and remeasure deviation.

12. If no improvement, administer remainder of Tensilon (0.3 to 0.5 cc).

13. If still no improvement, Tensilon test is negative.

ADVERSE EFFECTS OF TENSILON

(These can be minimized by using atropine.)

- Bradycardia
- Hypotension
- Tearing
- Salivation
- Sweating
- Nausea
- Vomiting
- Fainting
- Involuntary defecation

21

Retrobulbar Anesthesia

INDICATIONS

For anesthesia and akinesia of the globe for various procedures
(ie, cataract surgery, retinal procedures).

EQUIPMENT

- 10-mL syringe
- 18-gauge needle
- Retrobulbar needle or 25-gauge needle $1^1/_4$-inches long
- 4 × 4 gauze
- Betadine swabs
- 2% lidocaine with 1:100,000 epinephrine
- 0.75% bupivacaine

TECHNIQUE

1. Assemble the necessary instruments and supplies.

2. Draw up a 50:50 mixture of 2% lidocaine with 1:100.000 epinephrine and 0.75% bupivacaine into a 10-mL syringe using the 18-gauge needle.
3. Replace the 18-gauge needle with the retrobulbar needle.
4. Clean the eye area. Divide the lower eye orbital rim into thirds and identify the spot at the lateral third and the medial two thirds (Fig. 21-1). Pass the needle transcutaneously or transconjunctivally at the identified spot so that the needle is parallel to the orbit floor and away from the globe. (Fig. 21-2). One may use the hand that is not holding the needle to push the globe superiorly to further avoid the needle.
5. When the needle passes the globe equator, direct the needle slightly upwards to enter the intraconal space as seen in the Fig. 21-3. Retract the plunger of the syringe to check for blood. Then inject 3 to 5 cc of the block.
6. Withdraw the needle and massage the globe with the 4 × 4 gauze to reduce retrobulbar hemorrhage.

NOTES

Always watch the globe during injection to look for signs of perforation or retrobulbar hemorrhage.

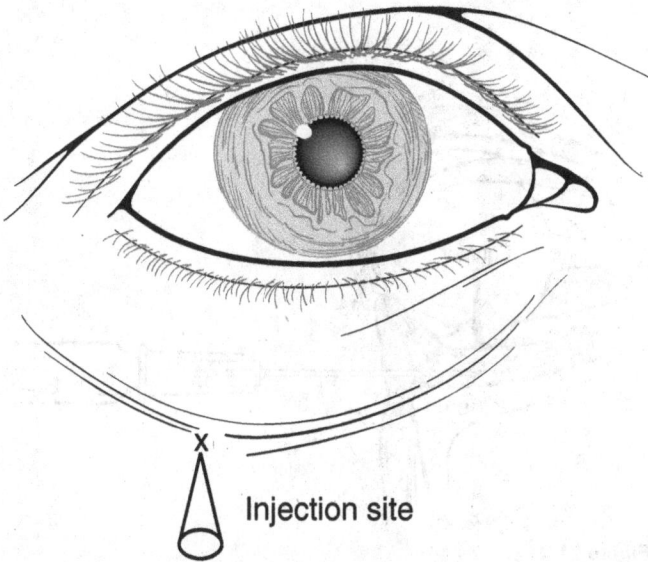

Injection site

Figure 21-1

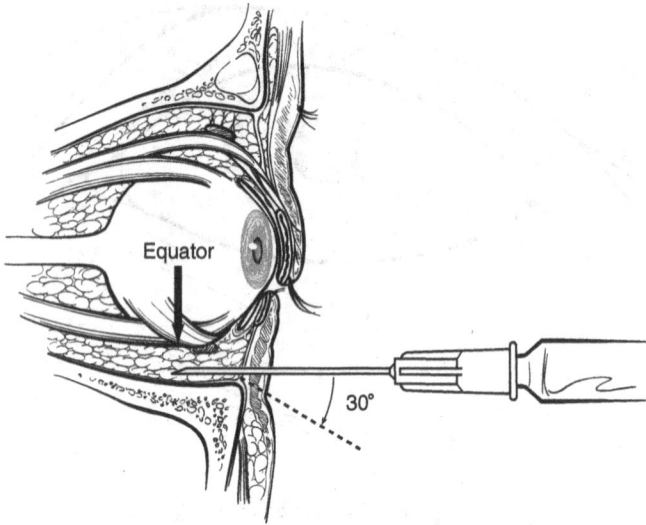

Equator

30°

Figure 21-2

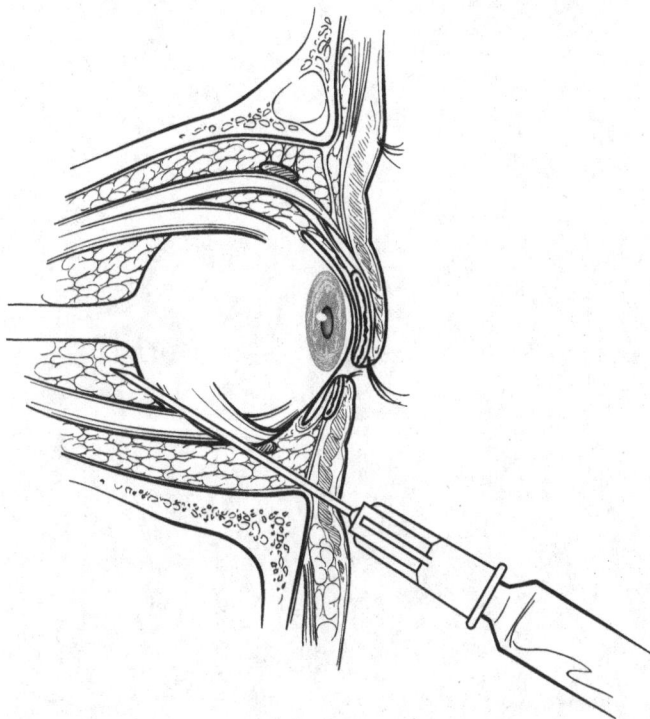

Figure 21-3

22

Forced Ductions

INDICATIONS

For differentiation of restrictive pattern motility disorders from paretic motility disorders.

EQUIPMENT

- Topical anesthetic (proparacaine or tetracaine drops)
- Sterile cotton tips
- Bishop forceps or equivalent
- 10% cocaine solution (optional)

TECHNIQUE

1. Place a drop of topical anesthetic into the eye being evaluated. Occasionally, placing a cotton-tipped applicator soaked in topical anesthetic or 10% cocaine for 1 to 2 minutes over the muscle insertion (Fig. 22-1) to be grasped is necessary for adequate anesthesia.
2. Grasp the muscle tendon in the field of gaze opposite the suspected restricted muscle (Fig. 22-2).

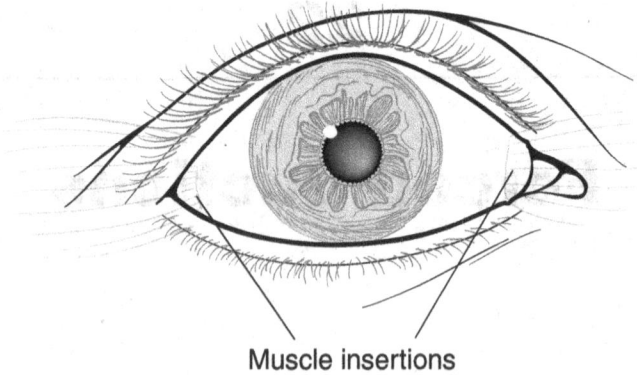

Muscle insertions

Figure 22-1

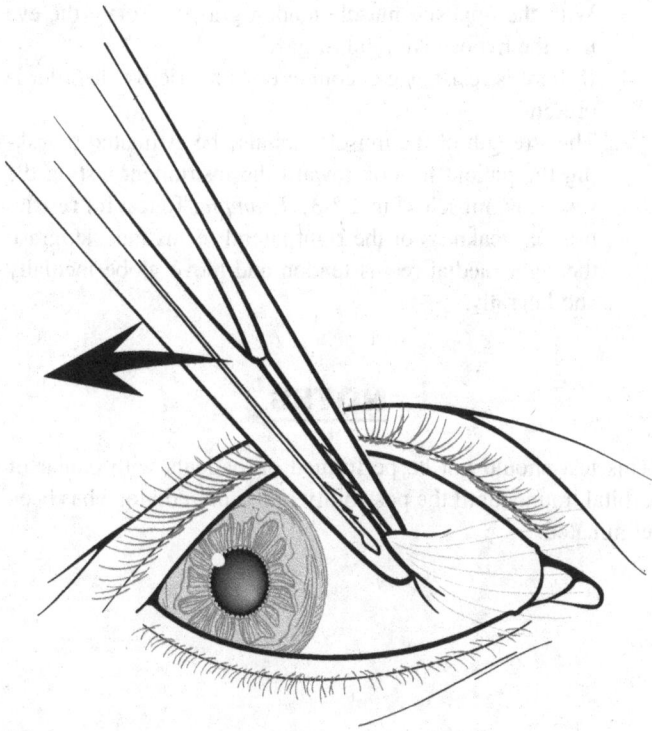

Figure 22-2

3. With the opposite muscle tendon grasped, rotate the eye into the hypoactive field of gaze.
4. If there is resistance encountered, a restrictive disorder is present.
5. The strength of the muscle can also be estimated by asking the patient to look toward the instrument testing the suspected muscle (Fig. 22-3). *Example*: To test for restriction or weakness of the right lateral rectus muscle, grasp the right medial rectus tendon and move globe medially and laterally.

NOTES

This test should not be performed on patients with ocular or orbital trauma until the possibility of a ruptured globe has been eliminated.

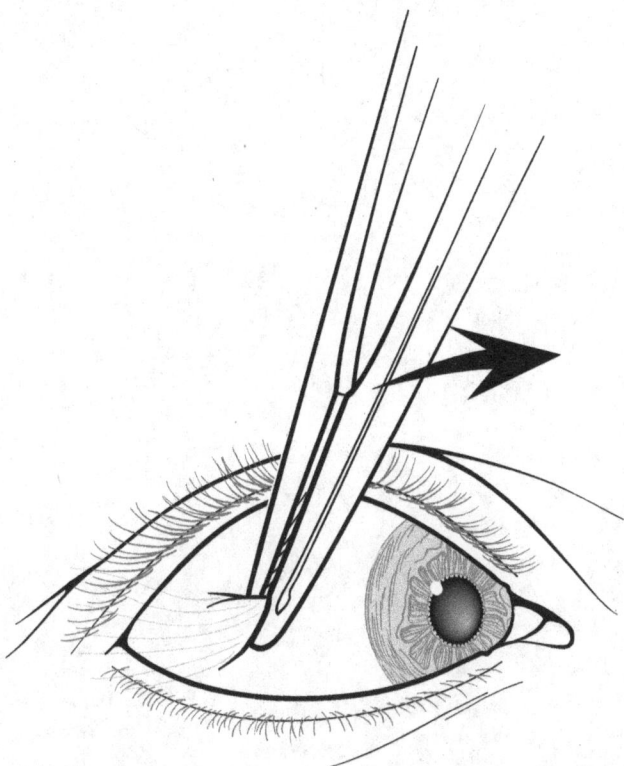

Figure 22-3

Part 5

Oculo-Plastics

23

Dye Disappearance Test

INDICATIONS

For evaluation of epiphora secondary to decreased nasolacrimal outflow.

EQUIPMENT

- Topical anesthetic (proparacaine or tetracaine drops)
- Fluorescein strip
- Watch or timer
- Cobalt blue light (on slit lamp or indirect ophthalmoscope)

TECHNIQUE

1. Assemble the necessary instruments and supplies.
2. Moisten the fluorescein strip with proparacaine and blot off the excess fluid.

2. Touch the strip to the inferior palpebral conjunctiva of each eye and make note of level of tear film (Fig. 23-1 top)
4. Wait 5 minutes.
5. Under blue light examination, examine for retention of fluorescein in the tear film. If fluorescein is still present after 5 minutes, this is a positive test and nasolacrimal duct insufficiency or obstruction exists. (Fig. 23-1 bottom).

NOTES

Occasionally, fluorescein will be seen remaining in the tear film of both eyes after 5 minutes, despite only symptomatic complaints from one eye. This finding is generally accompanied by a larger tear film meniscus of the symptomatic eye. This observation may be sufficient to conclude this test. Without this feature, the examination can be carried another 5 minutes more, when a discernable difference may be appreciated. In our experience, this is seldom necessary.

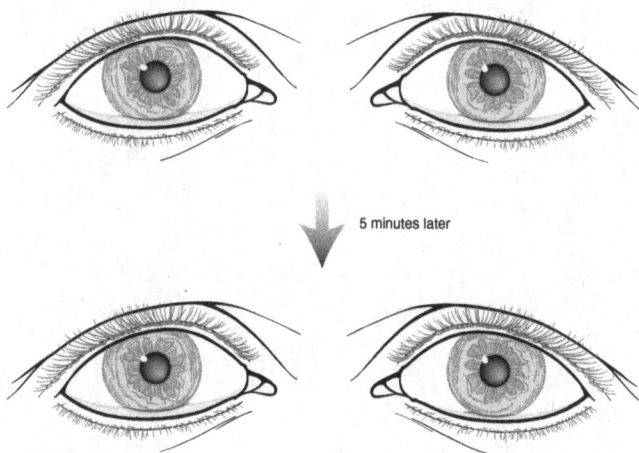

5 minutes later

Figure 23-1

24

Punctal Plug Insertion

INDICATIONS

For temporary occlusion of eyelid puncta.

EQUIPMENT

- Topical anesthetic (proparacaine or tetracaine drops)
- Punctal dilator
- Commercially available punctal plugs

TECHNIQUE

1. Assemble the necessary instruments and supplies.
2. Anesthetize the eye with several drops of topical anesthetic (proparacaine drops).
3. Have patient position comfortably in the slit lamp.
4. Estimate the size of the puncta and use the appropriate sized plug.
5. A dilator may be used to dilate the punctal opening prior to inserting the plug (Fig. 24-1).

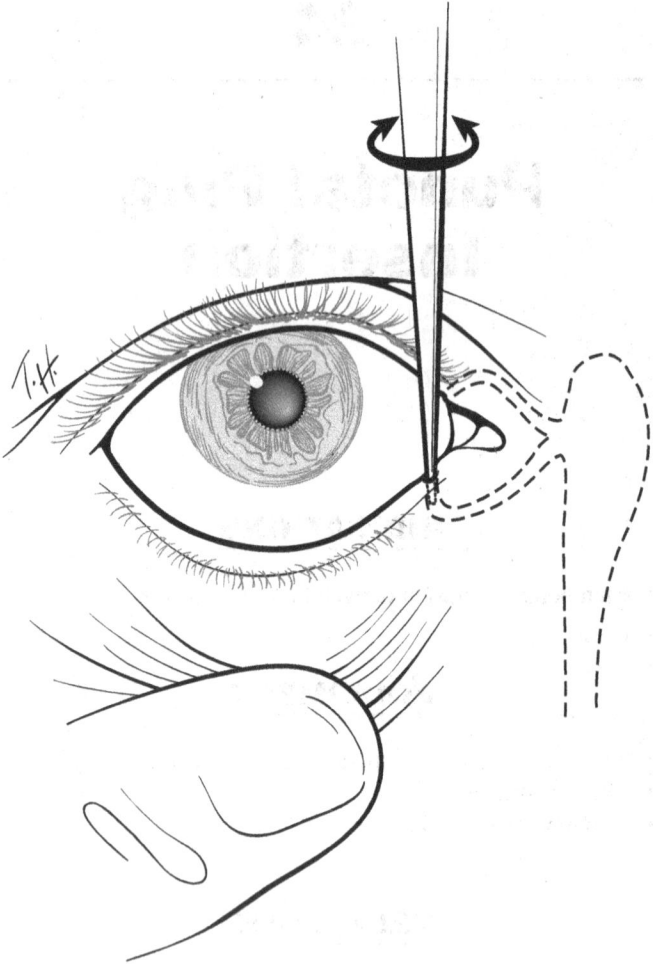

Figure 24-1

6. Evert the eyelid with lateral traction to better expose the puncta (Fig. 24-2).
7. Insert the plug dispenser into the puncta and insert the plug into the eye.
8. Examine for placement of the plug flush with the lid margin (Fig. 24-3).

NOTES

Punctal plugs are an excellent temporary means to alleviate the symptoms of dry eye. Care must be taken not to insert the plug too far into the canalicular system.

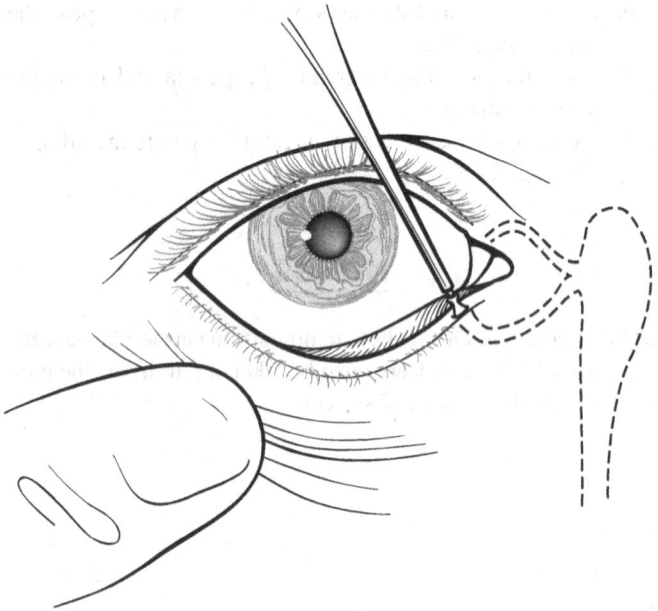

Figure 24-2

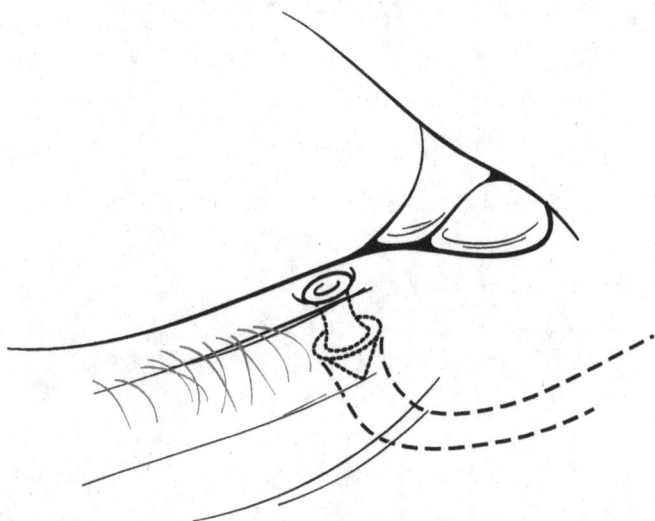

Figure 24-3

25

Permanent Punctal Occlusion

INDICATIONS

For permanent occlusion of eyelid puncta.

EQUIPMENT

- Topical anesthetic (proparacaine or tetracaine drops)
- Betadine swab
- 2% lidocaine with epinephrine in 3-cc syringe with 30-gauge needle
- Hemocautery
- Optional corneal shell
- Antibiotic ointment

TECHNIQUE

1. Assemble the necessary instruments and supplies.
2. Anesthetize the eye with several drops of topical anesthetic (proparacaine or tetracaine drops).

3. Swab the eyelid area with a Betadine swab or 75% alcohol prep pad.
4. With magnifying loupes or at the slit lamp, position the patient and locate the puncta.
5. Inject 0.5 cc of lidocaine into the skin around the punctum.
6. Evert the eyelid with lateral traction to better expose the punctum. Take the hemocautery and narrow the tip with your fingertips so that it will fit into the punctal opening.
7. To permanently seal the punctum, insert the cautery into the punctum 3 mm and in one maneuver, activate and slowly withdraw the cautery (Fig. 25-1a and 25-1b).
8. An alternative and less destructive method is to tap the top of the punctum with the activated cautery for 1 to 2 seconds to seal it.
9. Put antibiotic ointment in the eye.

NOTES

Always try punctal plugs prior to cauterization to evaluate for epiphora. Cauterization of one punctum per eye at a time will also minimize risk of epiphora as well.

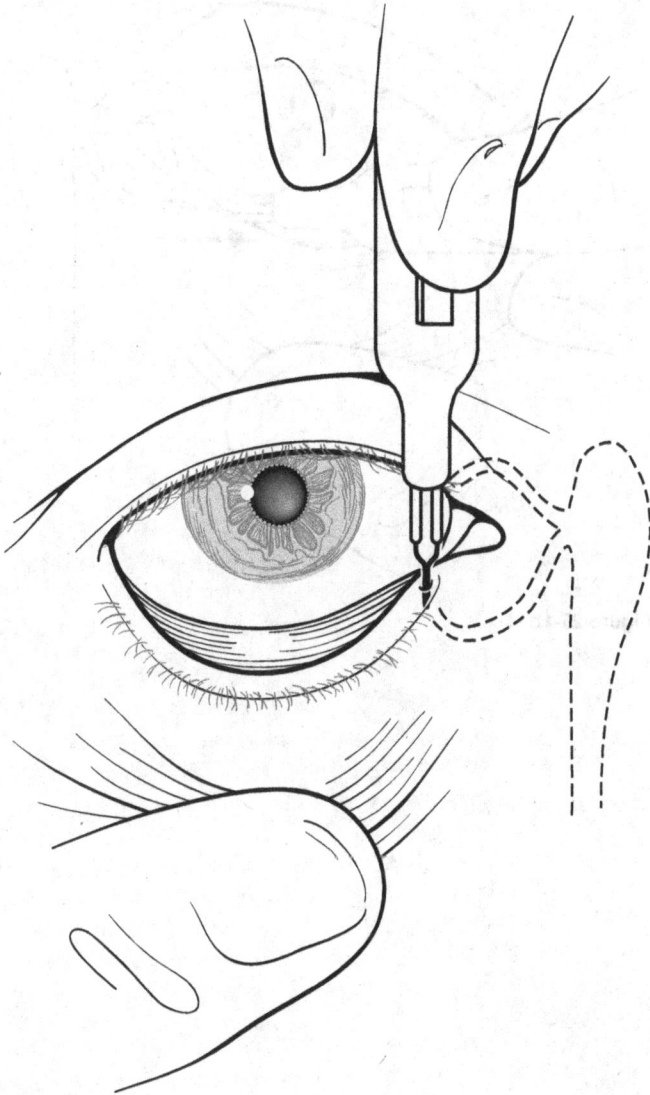

Figure 25-1a

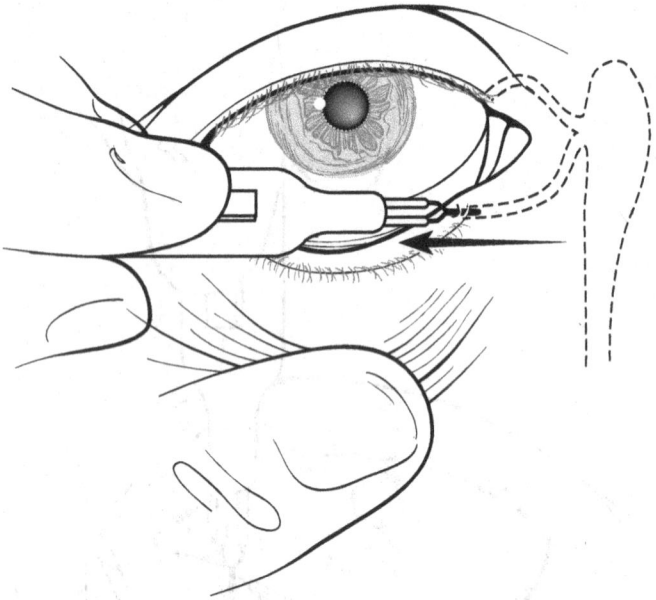

Figure 25-1b

26

Nasolacrimal Duct Obstruction Assessment/ Jones Testing

INDICATIONS

For the evaluation of tearing disorders associated with decreased nasolacrimal outflow.

TECHNIQUE

Equipment

- Moistened fluorescein strip
- Sterile cotton tips
- Watch or timer
- Saline flush on a 3- to 5-cc syringe
- Punctal dilator
- Lacrimal cannula

JONES I TEST

1. Place a moistened fluorescein strip onto the bulbar or palpebral conjunctival surface of the affected eye or eyes (Fig. 26-1).
2. Using a cotton-tipped applicator, place the tip near the ostium of the inferior meatus of the nose at both 2 and 5 minutes (Fig. 26-2).
3. If fluorescein is retrieved in the nose, this is a **positive** Jones test, and the nasolacrimal system is functioning appropriately (Table 26.1).
4. If no fluorescein is retrieved, there is either a physiologic dysfunction, an obstruction in the system, or a false-negative result.
5. Proceed with Jones II test.

NOTES

The Jones I test is not commonly used. It can give a false-negative result in up to one third of normal patients.

JONES II TEST

1. Have the patient tilt the head forward and irrigate the remaining fluorescein from the conjunctival fornix with saline.
2. Using the lacrimal cannula on a saline flush, introduce the lacrimal cannula into the inferior lacrimal puncta perpendicular to the lid margin. Rotate the cannula to the horizontal and advance along the canaliculus. (Fig. 26-3a and 26-3b).
3. Flush the nasolacrimal system with 0.5 to 1.0 cc of saline and observe for regurgitation of fluid from the same or opposite punctum.
4. Using the cotton-tipped applicator, attempt to retrieve fluorescein within the saline irrigation fluid at the ostium of the nasolacrimal duct in the inferior meatus.
5. If fluorescein is retrieved, this is a **positive** test.
6. If pt tastes saline, this is a negative test.

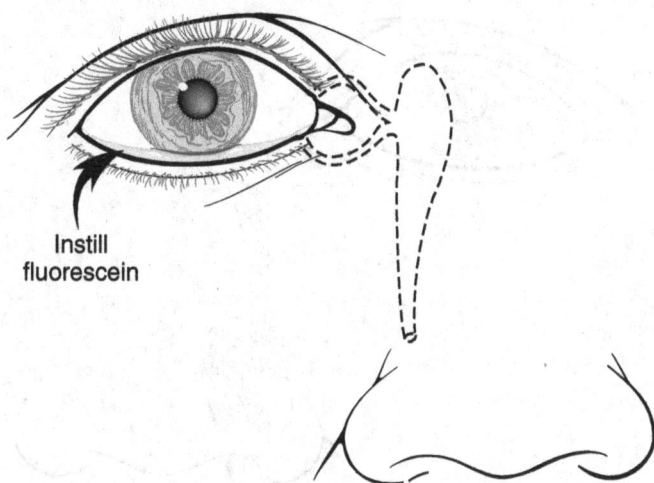

Instill
fluorescein

Figure 26-1

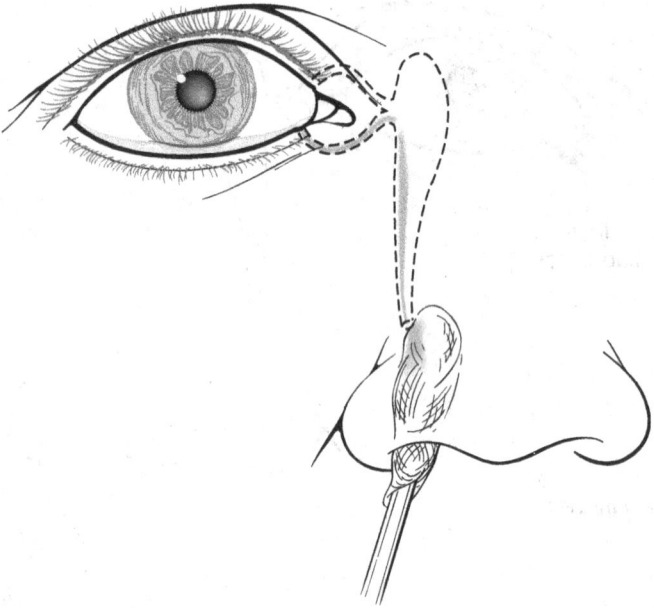

Figure 26-2

Table 26-1 Results of Jones Testing

Result	Interpretations
Jones I test	
Dye in nose	Patent system, probably normal physiologic function
No dye in nose	Physiologic dysfunction, anatomic obstruction, or false negative
Jones II test	
Dye in nose	Partial block of lower sac or duct
Saline in nose	Punctal or canalicular stenosis
Regurgitation at opposite puncta with dye	Complete nasolacrimal duct obstruction
Regurgitation at opposite puncta without dye	Complete common canaliculus obstruction
Regurgitation at same puncta with dye	Complete common canaliculus obstruction

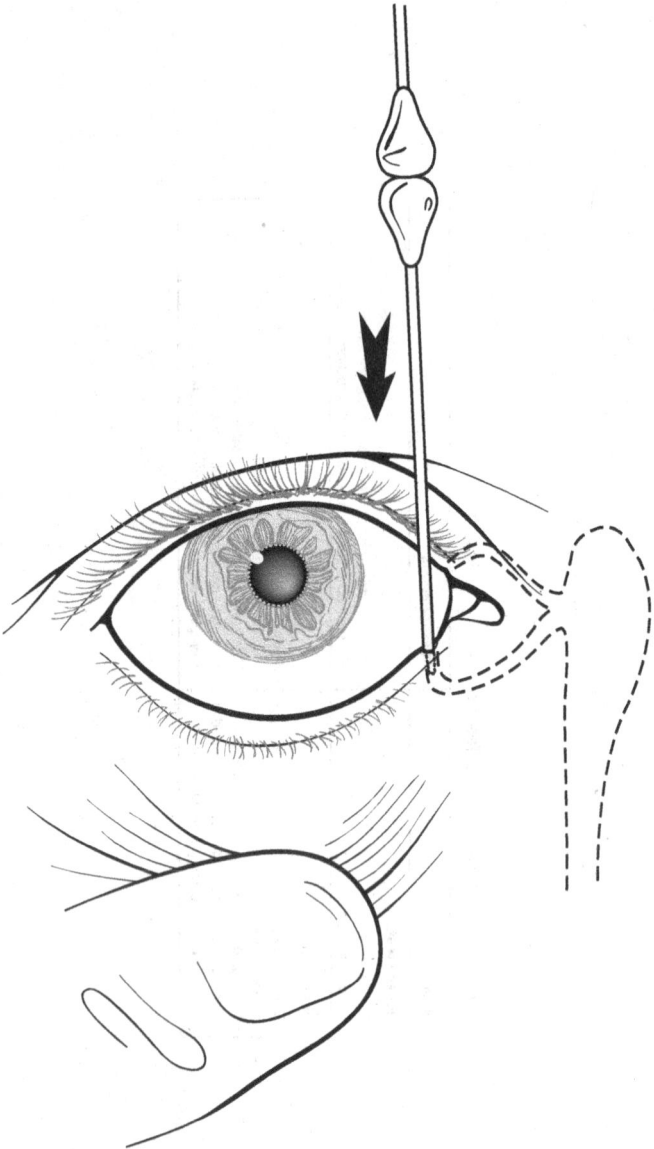

Figure 26-3a

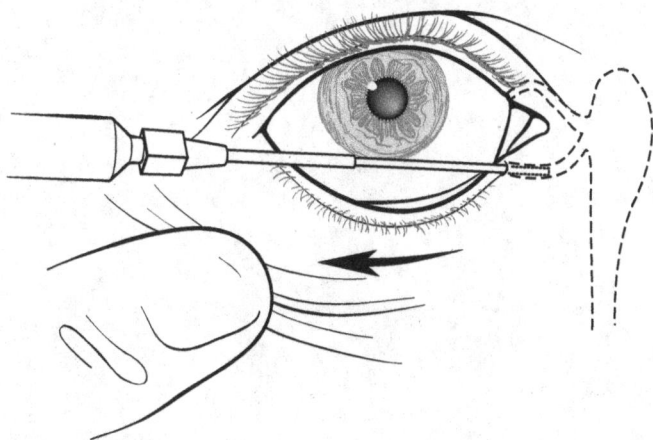

Figure 26-3b

27

Nasolacrimal Duct Probing

INDICATIONS

For tearing secondary to nasolacrimal duct obstruction in pediatric patients.

EQUIPMENT

- Topical anesthetic (proparacaine or tetracaine drops)
- Punctal dilator
- Bowman Probe (no. 00, 0, 1, or 2)
- 3-cc syringe
- Lacrimal cannula tip
- Saline solution
- Magnifying loupes (optional)
- Antibiotic ointment (erythromycin or bacitracin)

TECHNIQUE

1. Assemble the necessary instruments and supplies.
2. Anesthetize the eye with several drops of topical anesthetic (proparacaine or tetracaine drops).

3. With magnifying loupes, position the patient and identify the superior punctum.
4. Use the punctal dilator to enter the punctum. Then angle the dilator slightly downward toward the lid margin inside the canaliculus while putting traction on the lateral lid margin (Fig. 27-1). Remove punctal dilator.
5. Use a no. 0 or 00 Bowman probe to pass through the punctum into the canaliculus until reaching a hard stop. Be sure to apply lateral traction to the lateral lid margin and angle the probe slightly downward until a hard stop is reached. The hard stop is the edge of the bony naso-lacrimal sac.
6. Rotate the probe in a flat plane downward into the naso-lacrimal duct. The curved end of the probe should point posteriorly.
7. Advance the probe gently; there should not be any significant resistance (Fig. 27-2).
8. Remove the probe.
9. Instill 1 cc of saline solution into the upper puncta. Beware of overirrigation, which may cause laryngospasm. The fluid should flow freely through the nasolacrimal duct into the nose. If there is regurgitation of fluid or high pressure is required, consider repeating the probing. If after two attempts the probing is still unsuccessful, consider dacryocystorhinostomy.
9. Instill antibiotic ointment.

NOTES

This procedure is often done under masked general anesthesia in children. During the probing, one will often feel a membrane pop or resistance from a narrowed nasolacrimal duct. It is important to record this in the operation note. Beware of false passages.

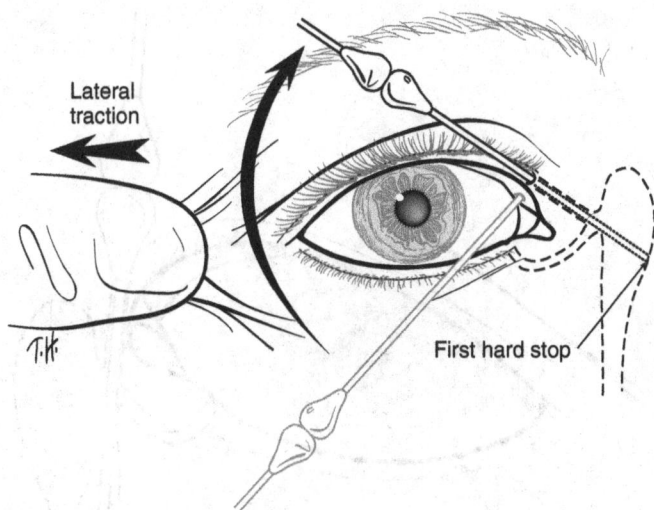

Figure 27-1

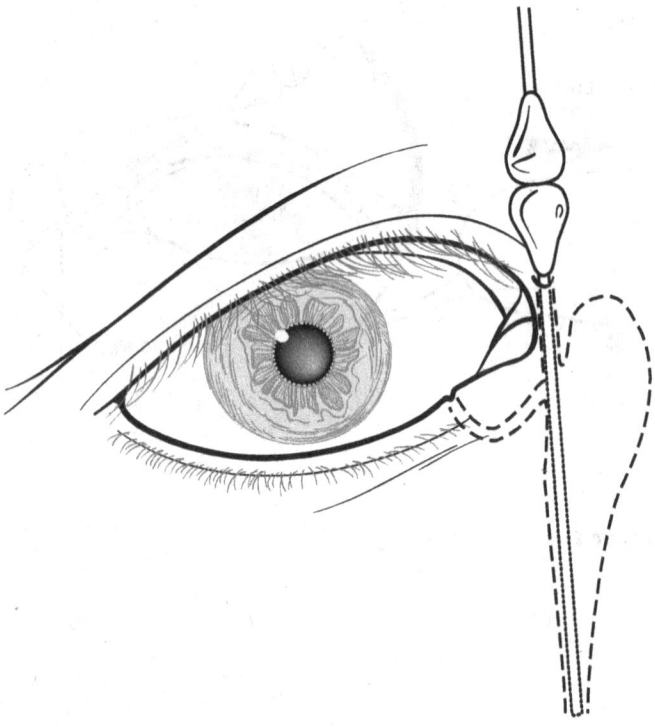

Figure 27-2

28

Phenylephrine Test

INDICATIONS

To evaluate for ptosis in unilateral or asymmetric acquired ptosis or to assess Mueller muscle activity in relation to ptosis.

EQUIPMENT

- Ruler
- Phenylephrine 2.5% drops

TECHNIQUE

1. Assemble the necessary instruments and supplies.
2. Measure lid-to-pupil distance as seen in Fig. 28-1. Also evaluate levator function by measuring excursion of upper lid from down- to upgaze (Fig. 28-2).
3. Instill phenylephrine 2.5% into the ptotic eye. Wait 10 minutes. If the ptotic lid is elevated to the desired lid height or >3 mm from baseline, then correction of ptosis may be aided by Mueller muscle resection.

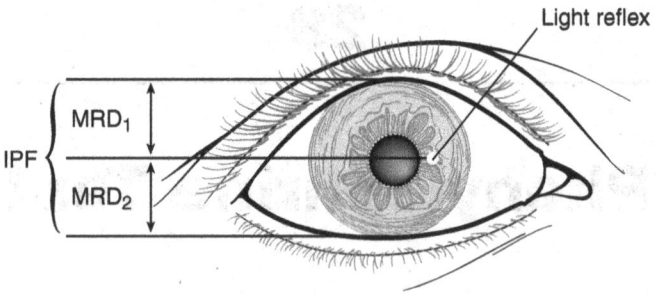

MRD$_1$ = Margin-Reflex Distance 1
MRD$_2$ = Margin-Reflex Distance 2
IPF = Interpal Pebral Fissure

Figure 28-1

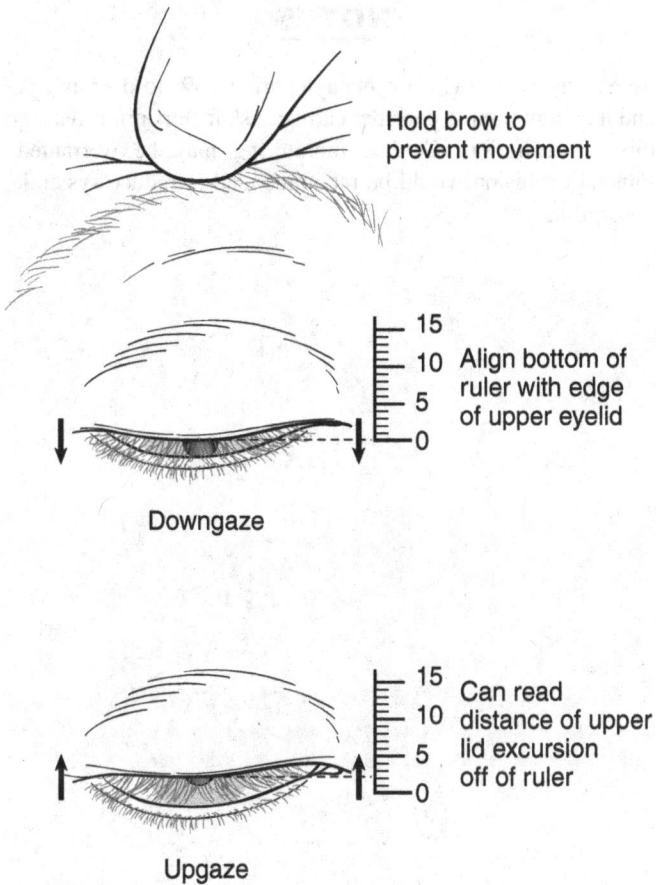

Hold brow to prevent movement

15
10
5
0

Align bottom of ruler with edge of upper eyelid

Downgaze

15
10
5
0

Can read distance of upper lid excursion off of ruler

Upgaze

Figure 28-2

NOTES

Some physicians will use phenylephrine 10% to do this test, and it is important to consider cardiac risk factors prior to using this concentration. Cardiac monitoring may be warranted. Punctal occlusion would be recommended to reduce systemic absorption.

29

Eyelid Laceration Repair Not Involving Lid Margin

INDICATIONS

To repair small eyelid lacerations in an office or emergency room setting. Avoid using the following technique for repairs involving large skin defects, severe distortion of the lid anatomy, damage to the lacrimal drainage apparatus, and lacerations associated with a ruptured globe.

EQUIPMENT

- 2% Lidocaine with 1:100,000 epinephrine
- 5-cc syringe
- 18-gauge and 30-gauge needles
- Lid laceration repair kit
- Fine-toothed Bishop Harmon forceps
- Castroviejo ophthalmic needle holder
- Straight Stevens scissors
- Skin retractors
- 6-0 Vicryl and 6-0 nylon suture

TECHNIQUE

1. Determine the extent of the injury. Complete the eye examination including the dilated fundus exam and computed tomography (CT) scan. Consider tetanus prophylaxis.
2. Assemble the necessary instruments and supplies.
3. Clean and irrigate the area of injury with saline. Identify and remove foreign bodies. Avoid tissue débridement. The face is well vascularized and responds well to repair. Once tissue is removed, it is often difficult to replace.
4. Administer local subcutaneous anesthetic to the wound site using the 30-gauge needle. Use Betadine swabs to clean the skin and surrounding areas.
5. Close the wound in layers, suturing the deepest layers first. Use 5-0 or 6-0 Vicryl suture for deep interrupted sutures (Fig. 29-1). The subcutaneous layers are the most important for maintaining skin tension and achieving good wound closure. Well placed subcutaneous sutures are important for having an aesthetically pleasing repair.
6. For the skin closure, one can use 6-0 Prolene or nylon suture in interrupted or subcuticular technique for skin closure of the eyelid. In areas of high tension (such as the eyebrow or forehead) use vertical mattress sutures. Consider using 6-0 fast-absorbing gut for wound closure in children or in patients who may not return for suture removal.
7. If orbital fat or significant ptosis is present, there is a high possibility of levator involvement. In general, orbital fat requires good hemostasis using hemocautery or a bipolar cautery. In many cases, it is better to not attempt to fix the levator on primary repair. The levator may best be repaired many months later.
8. Apply erythromycin ointment to the wound. Patients should return in 1 week for suture removal.

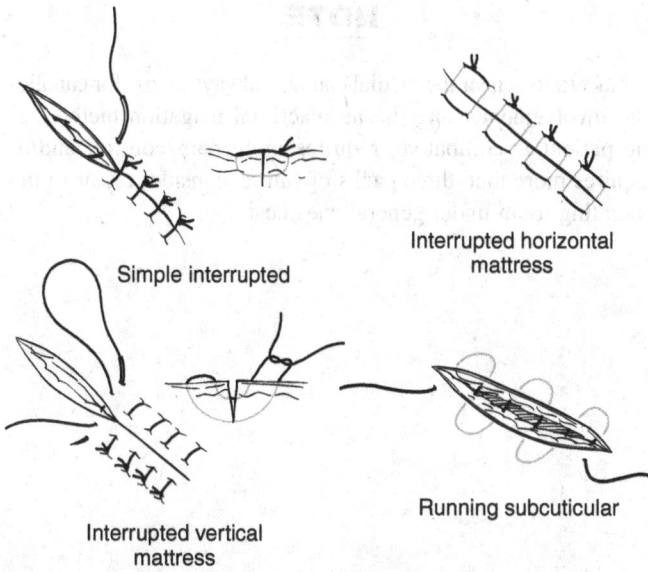

Simple interrupted

Interrupted horizontal
mattress

Interrupted vertical
mattress

Running subcuticular

Figure 29-1

NOTE

For lacerations near the medial canthus, always assess for canalicular involvement using the nasolacrimal irrigation method. If the patient is combative, requires more pain control, and/or requires more than three packs of suture, consider repair in the operating room under general anesthesia.

30

Eyelid Laceration Repair Involving Lid Margin

INDICATIONS

For eyelid lacerations at the lid margins without large defect or skin loss, i.e. closure with less than 25% tissue loss.

EQUIPMENT

- Proparacaine
- 5-cc syringe
- 18-gauge and 30-gauge needles
- Lid laceration repair kit
- Topical proparacaine
- Corneal shield
- Fine-toothed Bishop Harmon forceps
- Castroviejo ophthalmic needle holder
- Suture scissors
- 6-0 Silk and 6-0 Vicryl suture
- Magnifying loupes
- Antibiotic ointment (erythromycin or bacitracin)

TECHNIQUE

1. Assemble the necessary instruments and supplies.
2. Anesthetize the eye with several drops of topical proparacaine.
3. Place the corneal shield into the eye.
4. All lid margin sutures require silk suture to avoid abrading the cornea. Use 6-0 silk for a vertical mattress suture posterior to the meibomian gland orifices (Fig. 30-1).
5. Use 6-0 Vicryl for interrupted subcutaneous sutures along the length of the laceration and partial thickness through the tarsus. Make sure these sutures do not pass through the full thickness of the lid, or the sutures will rub against the eye (Fig. 30-2).
6. Place the second suture anterior to the gray line. Tie these sutures and leave the ends long. (Fig. 30-3). The key to the whole repair is precise reapproximation along the eyelid margin.
7. When tying the suture closest to the lid margin, tuck the lid sutures into the knot of the skin suture.

NOTES

If the laceration is near the medial third of the eyelid, always assess for canalicular laceration. These need to be repaired in the operating room immediately. Large eyelid lacerations with tissue loss should be fixed in the operating room, particularly when there is difficulty reapproximating the lid margin.

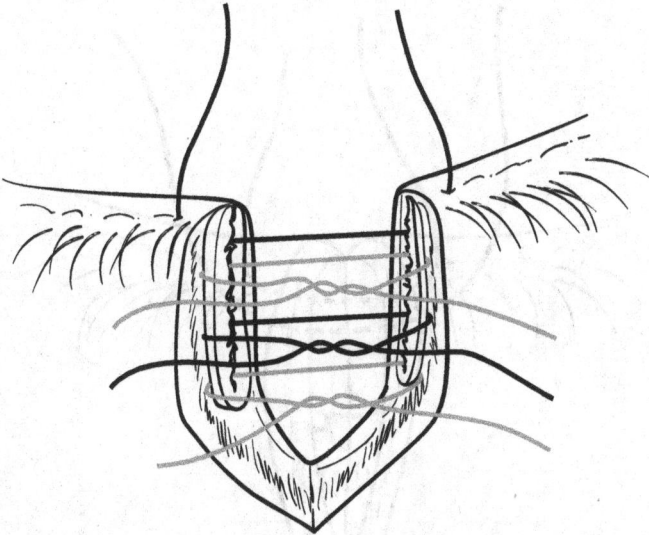

Figure 30-1

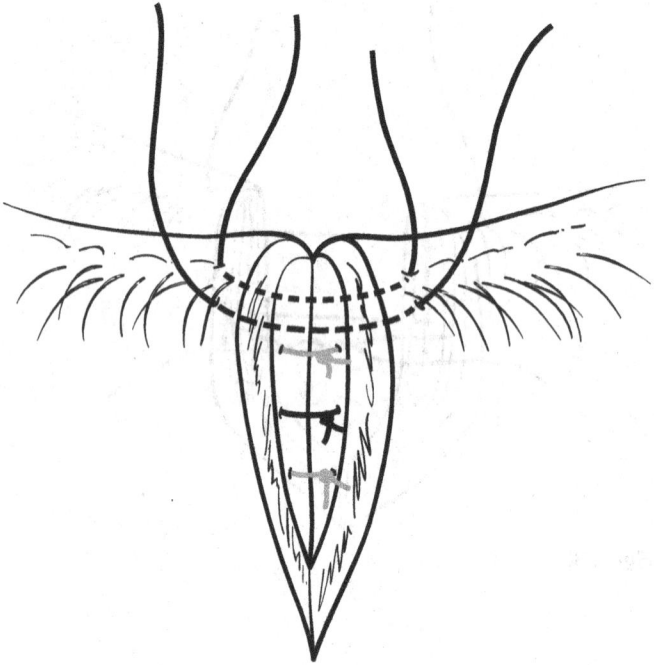

Figure 30-2

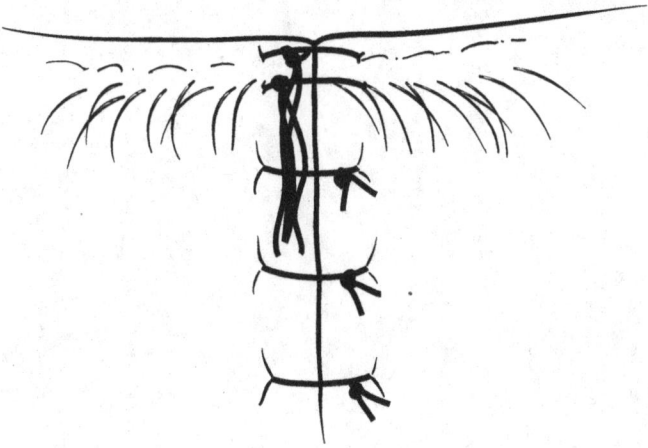

Figure 30-3

31

Canalicular Laceration Assessment

INDICATIONS

To assess for canaliculus damage in lacerations near the medial canthus.

EQUIPMENT

- Topical anesthetic (proparacaine or tetracaine drops)
- Punctal dilator
- 3-cc syringe
- Bowman probe (0 or 00)
- Lacrimal cannula tip
- Pigtail probe
- Saline solution
- Magnifying loupes (optional)
- Antibiotic ointment (erythromycin or bacitracin)

TECHNIQUE

1. Assemble the necessary instruments and supplies.
2. Anesthetize the eye with several drops of topical anesthetic.
3. With magnifying loupes, identify the superior puncta.
4. Use the punctal dilator to enter the puncta, then rotate the dilator laterally toward the lid margin while putting traction on the lateral lid margin (Figs. 31-1 and 31-2). Remove punctal dilator.
5. Insert the lacrimal cannula attached to the saline syringe in a similar fashion.
6. Instill 1 cc of saline solution into the lower punctum. Beware of overirrigation, which may cause laryngospasm. The fluid should flow freely down the nasolacrimal duct and either down the nose or the throat.
7. Observe any reflux of fluid (indicating nasolacrimal system obstruction) or flow of colored saline from the lacerated end of the canaliculus.
8. If canalicular laceration is present, insert the Bowman probe through the lower punctum to identify the proximal end of the laceration. The distal canaliculus can be difficult to identify. A pigtail probe inserted through the intact upper punctum can identify the other end of the lacerated canaliculus. This procedure is best done under anesthesia.
9. Repeat the above procedure for the upper canaliculus as well.

NOTES

Any laceration involving the eyelid near the puncta should be irrigated to assess for canalicular damage. These injuries must be repaired in the operating room, usually within 12 to 24 hours for best results.

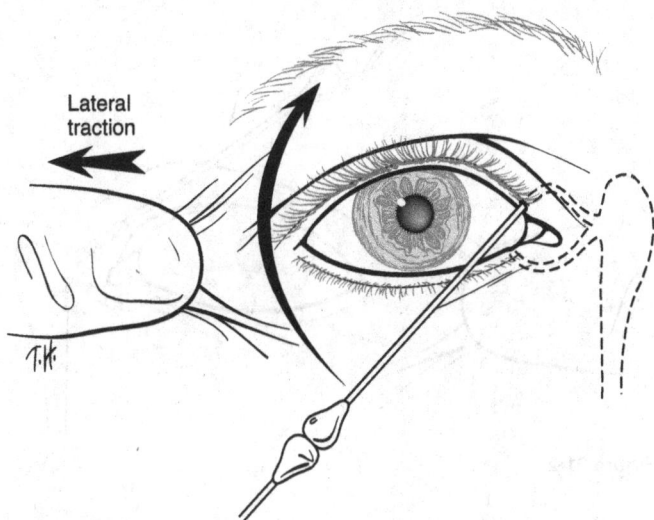

Figure 31-1

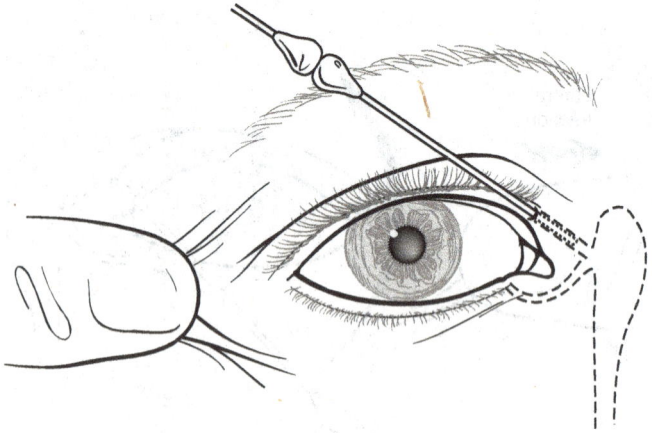

Figure 31-2

32

Removal of Benign Skin Lesion

INDICATIONS

For removal of benign skin lesions less than 1 cm in size around the eye.

EQUIPMENT

- 3-cc syringe
- 25-gauge needle
- 2% lidocaine with epinephrine
- Skin marking pen
- No. 15 Bard Parker blade
- Westcott scissors
- 0.3 Cassie forceps
- Needle holder
- Suture
- Steri-strips

TECHNIQUE

1. Draw an elliptical excision pattern around the skin lesion following the wrinkle pattern and skin contour lines.
2. Anesthetize the skin using the lidocaine.
3. With the no. 15 blade, incise the superficial skin along the marked path (Fig. 32-1).
4. Starting at one end of the lesion, lift up the skin and use the scissors to dissect a plane between the skin and subcutaneous tissue.
5. Small lesions can be reappoximated using a Steristrip
6. Larger lesions can be closed using interrupted sutures or a running subcuticular suture (Figs. 32-2 and 32-3).

NOTES

Malignant lesions may need wider or deeper excisions with specimens taken for examination using frozen section. Larger lesion removal may require skin grafting.

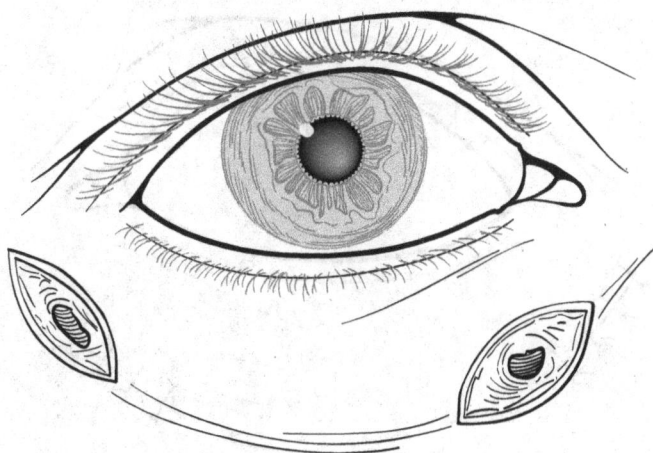

Figure 32-1

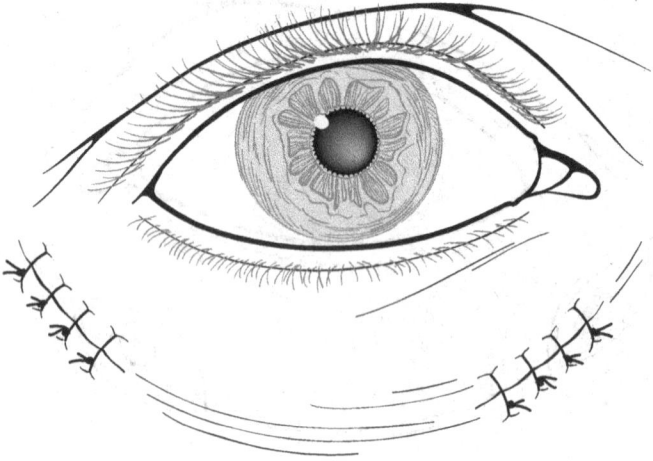

Figure 32-2

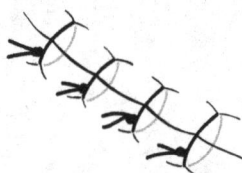

Interrupted suture

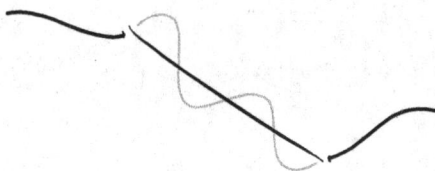

Running subcuticular
suture

Figure 32-3

33

Lateral Canthotomy and Cantholysis

INDICATIONS

For use in retrobulbar hemorrhage where ocular blood flow is compromised after medical measures as part of ectropion/ entropion repairs.

EQUIPMENT

- 30-gauge straight needle
- 1- to 3-cc syringe
- Lidocaine 2% with epinephrine
- Betadine 5% solution
- Topical proparacaine
- Hemostat
- Blunt tip Stevens scissors
- Bishop Harmon forceps
- Cotton-tipped applicators
- Sterile 4 × 4 gauze pads
- Sterile drape
- Sterile gloves
- Tape

TECHNIQUE FOR LATERAL CANTHOTOMY AND CANTHOLYSIS IN RETROBULBAR HEMORRHAGE

1. Place a drop of topical proparacaine onto the affected eye.
2. Prepare the surgical field with Betadine 5% and a sterile drape.
3. Inject the lateral canthal region with lidocaine 2% with epinephrine. Inject 1 to 2 mL and include the lateral orbital rim.
4. After anesthesia is obtained, place a hemostat across the lateral canthal angle, extending about 1 cm laterally and hold for 1 minute (Fig. 33-1).
5. Remove the hemostat and cut through the skin with the scalpel or scissors in the trough compressed earlier by the hemostat (Fig. 33-2). The globe may proptose somewhat from this maneuver. Use sterile cotton tips and gauze 4 × 4s for hemostasis if necessary.
6. The eyelids should move freely against the globe. Frequently, a lateral canthotomy is all that is necessary to allow the eye to perfuse adequately. If the eyelids are still tight and difficult to move digitally, a lateral cantholysis should also be performed.
7. Using the scissors, strum for the lateral canthal tendon by pointing the tips of the scissors towards the tip of the patient's nose and cut the tendon. The eye may proptose even more than previously (Fig. 33-3).
8. If visual acuity is still threatened, intraocular pressure is still elevated, or if color vision deteriorates, surgical orbital decompression may be necessary.
9. If adequately managed, place a sterile dressing over the wound, start oral antibiotics, and reassess daily until stable.
10. The wound can be repaired when the retrobulbar hemorrhage has resolved. In many cases, the lateral canthus will heal without need for revision.

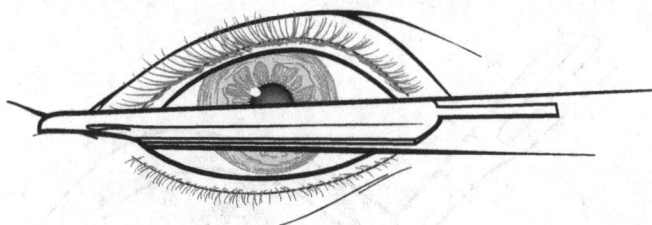

Figure 33-1

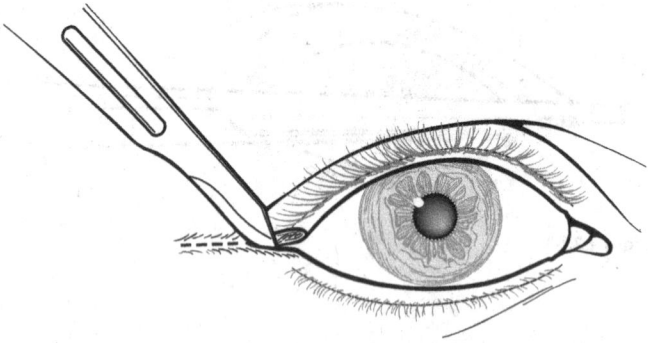

Figure 33-2

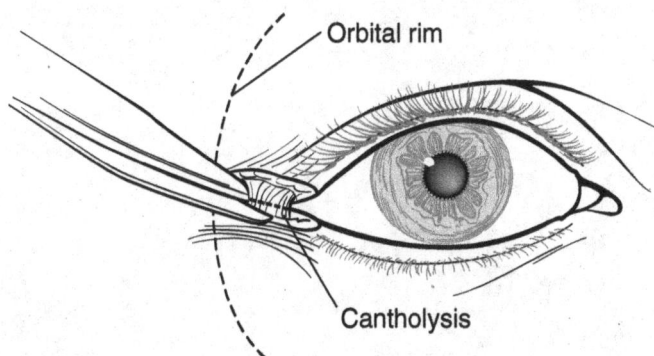

Figure 33-3

34

Suture Tarsorrhaphy (Frost Suture)

INDICATIONS

For temporary eyelid closure necessitated by ocular surface disease or ulceration. Closure of the lid often promotes surface healing by reducing drying, mechanical irritation, and exposure to the environment.

EQUIPMENT

- 30-gauge straight needle
- 1- to 3-cc syringe
- Lidocaine 2% with epinephrine
- Betadine 5% solution
- Topical proparacaine
- Westcott scissors
- Bishop Harmon forceps
- Needle holder
- Suture scissors

- 8-0 Nylon suture, double armed or 6-0 Prolene suture, double armed styrofoam suture packing for bolsters (or silicone from scleral buckle)
- Cotton-tipped applicators
- Sterile 4 × 4 gauze pads
- Sterile drape
- Sterile gloves
- Topical antibiotic

TECHNIQUE FOR SUTURE TARSORRHAPHY

1. Place a drop of topical proparacaine into the affected eye.
2. Place a drop of topical antibiotic into the affected eye.
3. Mark the lid margin indicating the location of the area of suture closure. Often, closing the lateral third of the eyelid provides excellent ocular protection and also allows examination of the ocular surface medially.
4. Prepare the surgical field with Betadine 5% and a sterile drape.
5. Inject the superior and inferior lids with lidocaine 2% near the lid margins in the area where the tarsorrhaphy is going to be placed.
6. Cut two small rectangular pieces of styrofoam from the suture packaging to use as suture bolsters.
7. Pass each end of the double armed 8-0 nylon through one of the bolsters.
8. Pass each end of the 8-0 nylon suture through the upper lid skin 2 to 3 mm superior to the lid margin with a bite of the tarsal plate, and exit the lid margin through the gray line (Fig. 34-1).
9. Pass each end of the 8-0 nylon suture through the lower lid margin gray line and exit the skin 2 to 3 mm inferior to the lid margin.
10. Again, pass each end of the double armed 8-0 nylon through the other bolster, tighten the suture, and tie it to approximate the lid margin in the desired position (Fig. 34-2).
11. These steps can be repeated if further eyelid closure is necessary.

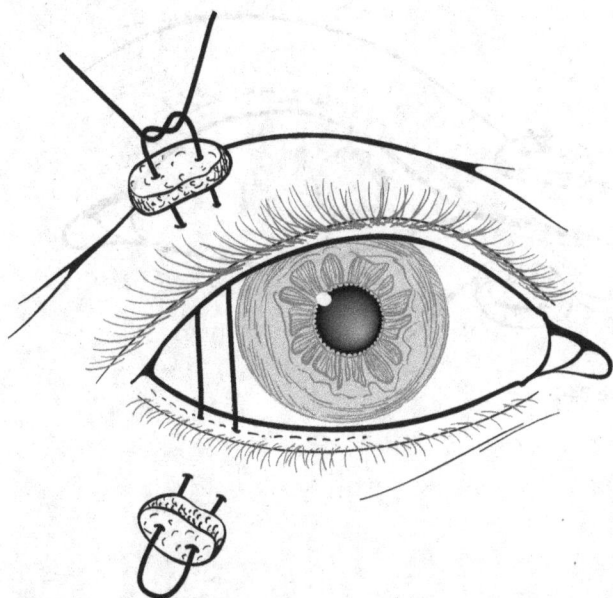

Figure 34-1

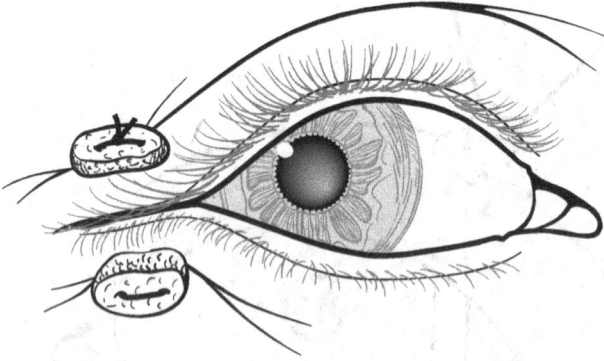

Figure 34-2

<u>NOTE</u>

For a more permanent eyelid closure, the epithelium of the gray line of the upper and lower eyelid margins can be excised. This permits adhesion of these two surfaces, which can keep the eyelid closed even after the nylon suture is removed.

35

Cilia (Eyelash) Removal

INDICATIONS

Ocular surface irritation may result from corneal or conjunctival contact with cilia. The following conditions may bring cilia
into contact with the globe.

- Distichiais: cilia protrude abnormally from meibomian
  glands
- Trichiasis: cilia originate from pretarsal skin (normal location) but are directed posteriorly
- Entropion: posterior rotation of entire lid margin directs
  cilia posteriorly
- Epiblepharon: fold of pretarsal skin pushes normal cilia
  posteriorly

EPILATION

Equipment

- Jeweler's forceps

Technique

1. Place the patient in the seated position in the slit lamp chair.
2. Hold the eyelid to rotate the lashes away from the globe.
3. Remove the cilia by grasping them at the base with the jeweler's forceps so as to remove the entire cilia without breaking it off above the base (Fig. 35-1).
4. Instruct the patient to return in 2 to 3 weeks for evaluation of cilia regrowth.

ELECTROLYSIS

Equipment

* Proparacaine eye drops
* Alcohol or iodine solution swab
* Lidocaine 2% with epinephrine
* 3-cc syringe
* 30-gauge hypodermic needle
* Hyfrecator
* Hyfrecator needle
* Jeweler's forceps

Technique

1. Draw up in a 3-cc syringe 3 mL of lidocaine 2% with epinephrine on a 30-gauge needle.
2. Place the patient in the examination chair and fully recline the chair.
3. Instill a drop of proparacaine into the operative eye, swab the lateral periorbital skin with alcohol or iodine solution and locally infiltrate or place a partial (upper lid or lower lid) van Lint block with lidocaine.

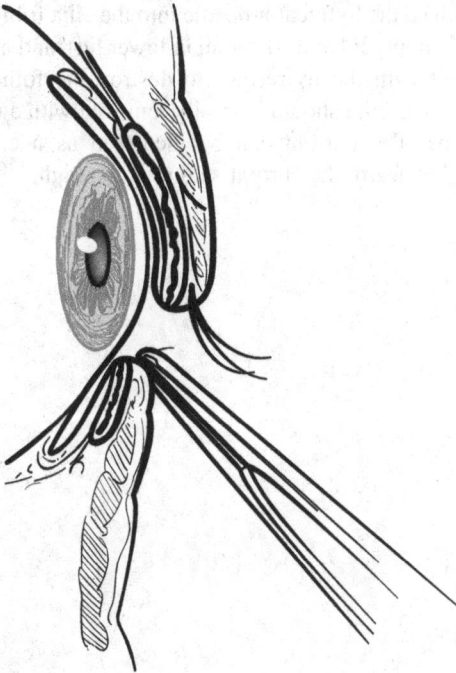

Figure 35-1

4. Introduce the hyfrecator needle into the cilia follicle (~2.5 mm in upper lid and ~1.5 mm in lower lid), and apply low current with the hyfrecator to destroy the follicle (Fig. 35-2). The cilia should be easily removed with a jeweler's forceps. The current can be increased as needed. If a "pop" is heard, the current setting is too high.

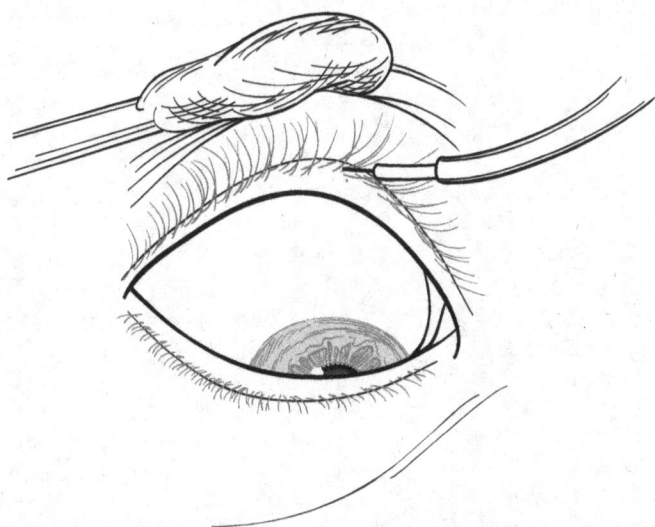

Figure 35-2

36

Quickert Sutures

INDICATIONS

Quickert sutures are used to temporarily repair lower lid entropion (Fig. 36-1). The plain gut sutures elicit a greater inflammatory response and scarring, which hold the eyelid in place.

EQUIPMENT

- 30-gauge straight needle
- 1- to 3-cc syringe
- Lidocaine 2% with epinephrine
- Bctadine 5% solution
- Topical proparacaine
- Three packs of 6-0 Vicryl or plain gut suture, double armed
- Sterile gloves
- Sterile drape
- Castroviejo needle driver
- Bishop Harmon forceps or 0.3 Cassie toothed forceps
- Suture tying forceps
- Westcott scissors
- Topical antibiotic ointment
- Scleral shell

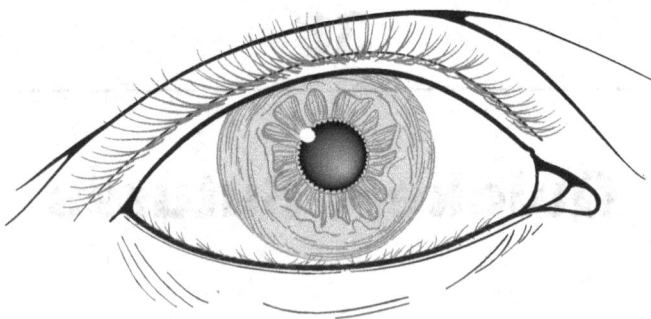

Figure 36-1

TECHNIQUE

1. Place a drop of topical proparacaine into the affected eye.
2. Place a drop of topical antibiotic into the affected eye.
3. Place a scleral shell into the eye.
4. Prepare the surgical field with Betadine 5% and a sterile drape.
5. Inject the lower eyelid with lidocaine 2% with epinephrine. Inject about 1 to 1.5 mL to provide adequate anesthesia for the entire lower lid.
6. Starting centrally on the lower eyelid, pass one arm of the 6-0 Vicryl suture through the inferior conjunctival fornix and aim the needle superiorly to exit the skin 1 to 2 mm inferior to the lash line. Do the same with the second arm of the suture approximately 2 to 3 mm laterally (Fig. 36-2).
7. Tie the suture just tight enough to gently evert the lashes away from the globe.
8. Repeat this procedure both nasally and temporally to the central stitch with the other Vicryl sutures.
9. Remove the scleral shell.
10. Place the patient on topical antibiotic ointment for 4 to 7 days.
11. These stitches generally last 2 to 4 weeks.

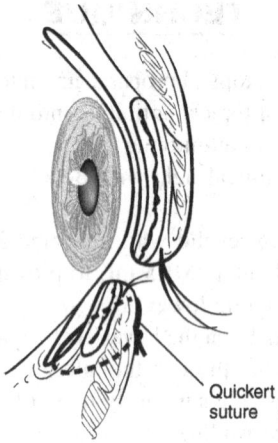

Quickert
suture

Figure 36-2

37

Punctoplasty

INDICATIONS

Punctal stenosis and epiphora (excessive tearing).

EQUIPMENT

- 2% Lidocaine with epinephrine
- 5% Povidone-iodine
- Syringe and 30-gauge needle
- Punctal dilator
- Sharp Westcott scissors
- Antibiotic-steroid ointment

TECHNIQUE

1. Assemble the necessary instruments and supplies.
2. Infiltrate eyelid with local anesthesia through 30-gauge needle.
3. Clean the eyelids with 5% povidone-iodine solution.
4. Evert the eyelid with the stenotic punctum.

5. Insert the punctal dilator to gently dilate the punctum. A sharp-tipped probe or sterile safety pin may be needed to open a completely stenotic punctum.
6. Insert one blade of the sharp Westcott scissors 2 to 3 mm into the punctum with the opposite blade on the conjunctival surface. Make a cut perpendicular to the eyelid margin (Fig. 37-1).
7. Make a second perpendicular cut starting approximately 1 mm from the first cut and connecting to the end of the first cut to excise a small triangular wedge of tissue.
8. Have the patient apply a combination antibiotic-steroid ointment to the eye twice a day for 5 days.

NOTES

Evaluate for nasolacrimal duct obstruction as a concomitant cause for tearing.

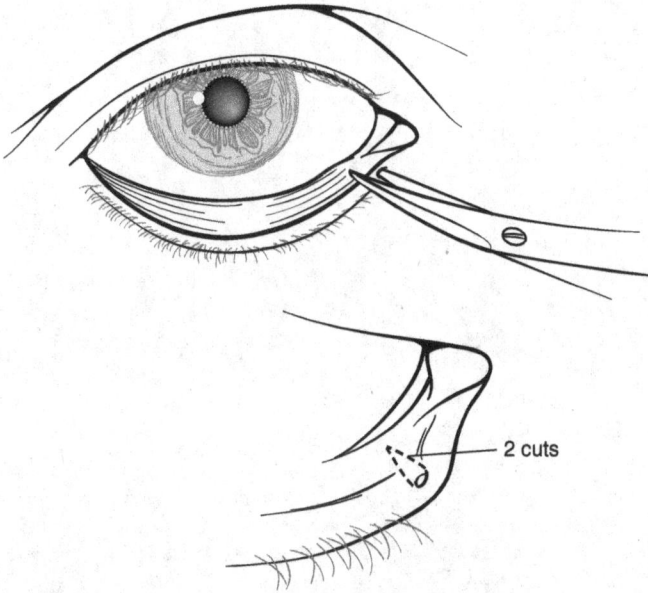

2 cuts

Figure 37-1

Part 6

Retina

Part 8

Poultry

38

Vitreous Tap/Intravitreal Antibiotic Injection

INDICATIONS

Bacterial endophthalmitis when therapeutic vitrectomy is not indicated.

EQUIPMENT

- Proparacaine or tetracaine anesthetic drops
- 5% Povidone-iodine
- 1-cc syringes
- 22- or 25-gauge needle
- 27-gauge needle
- Lid speculum
- Vancomycin 1 mg/0.1 mL
- Ceftazidime 2.25 mg/0.1 mL

TECHNIQUE

1. Assemble the necessary instruments and supplies.
2. Alert the microbiology lab to prepare for the vitreous specimen prior to the procedure.
3. Prep the eyelids with 5% povidone-iodine and place a drop in the conjunctival fornix.
4. Place the eyelid speculum in the eye. Anesthetize the eye with topical anesthetic drops.
5. Introduce a 22- or 25-gauge needle on a 1-cc syringe 3.5 to 4.0 mm posterior to the inferotemporal limbus and advance to the mid-vitreous cavity (Fig. 38-1).
6. Aspirate a 0.3-cc vitreous specimen.
7. Cap the syringe and transport to the microbiology lab for culture. If a lab is not available, the specimen may be directly inoculated into a blood culture bottle.
8. Inject 0.1 cc of vancomycin (1 mg/0.1 mL) using a 27-gauge needle on a 1-cc syringe through the pars plana. Repeat with ceftazidime (2.25 mg/0.1 mL).

NOTES

Dexamethasone 0.4 mg/0.1 mL can also be injected in addition to antibiotics to attempt to decrease inflammation. Vancomycin and ceftazidime are available as lyophilized powders, which are reconstituted with sterile water or normal saline. A portable battery-powered 23-gauge vitrector can be used as an alternative to obtain a larger vitreous sample through a self-sealing wound.

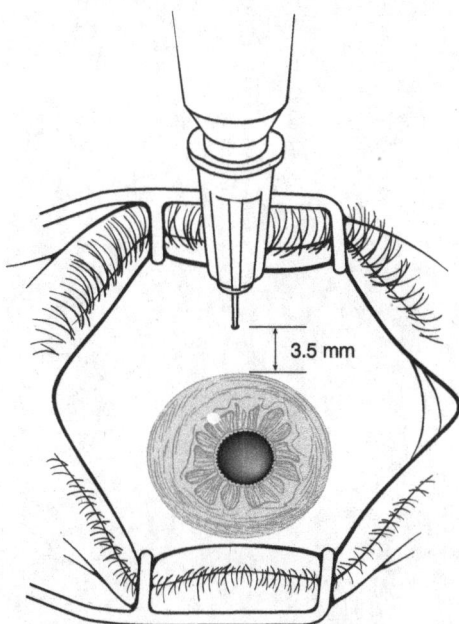

Figure 38-1

39

Panretinal Photocoagulation

INDICATIONS

High-risk proliferative retinopathy.

EQUIPMENT

- Contact lens
- Topical or retrobulbar anesthetic
- Coupling solution
- Argon laser

TECHNIQUE

1. Choose either topical or retrobulbar anesthesia based on the amount of treatment required and patient characteristics. Treatment may be started with topical anesthesia and changed to retrobulbar if the patient is very uncomfortable.
2. Place the contact lens of choice onto the selected eye with coupling solution. Ensure that there are no air bubbles (Fig. 39-1).

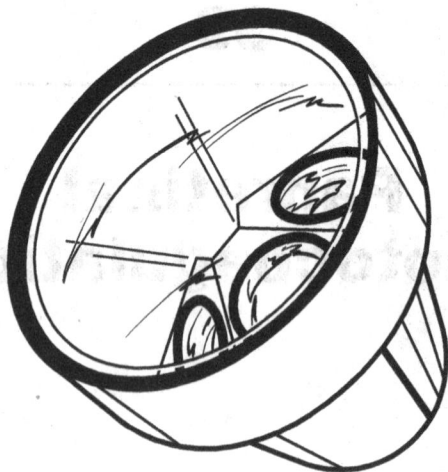

Figure 39-1

3. Use the following laser settings:
   - 500-μm spot size for Goldmann lens; 350-μm spot size for panfundoscopic lenses (ie, Rodenstock, Mainster, Quadraspheric)
   - Argon green wavelength
   - 0.1- to 0.2-second duration
   - 200 mW initial power
4. Focus the laser on the peripheral retina. Place a laser spot. Increase power as needed until a gray-white burn is visible.
5. Place gray-white burns one-half to one burn-width apart from the temporal arcades to anterior to the equator. Treat 2.5 to 3 disc diameters temporal to the fovea extending anteriorly. The area nasal to the disc can be treated to within one-half burn to one disc diameter, depending on the extent of neovascularization. Avoid the area of the posterior pole between the temporal arcades and disc extending to 2.5 disk diameters temporal to the fovea (Fig. 39-2).
6. Tailor treatment to the extent of neovascularization. Full panretinal photocoagulation (PRP) consists of 1200 or more burns. This can be divided into multiple sessions.
7. Our suggested method is to always place burns in a posterior-to-anterior direction to avoid inadvertent extension into the macula. Start with burns nasal to the disc and move segmentally into the inferior quadrants (Fig. 39-3). Place a double row of barrier burns 2.5 to 3 disk diameters temporal to the fovea. Then treat the area temporal to the barrier. Finally, treat the superior quadrants.

PITFALLS

- Advise the patient before the procedure that there may be a loss of peripheral and night vision. There may also be a loss of accommodation. Visual acuity may decrease 1 to 2 lines.
- PRP may worsen macular edema. If significant macular edema is present, focal laser treatment should be performed prior to PRP.

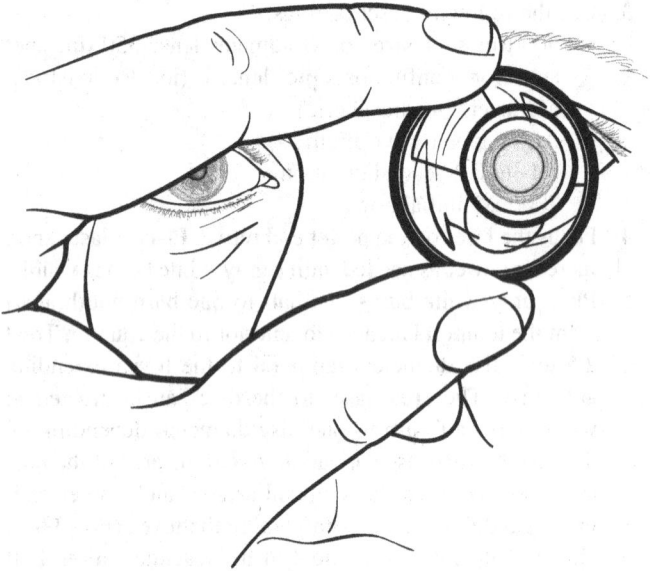

Figure 39-2

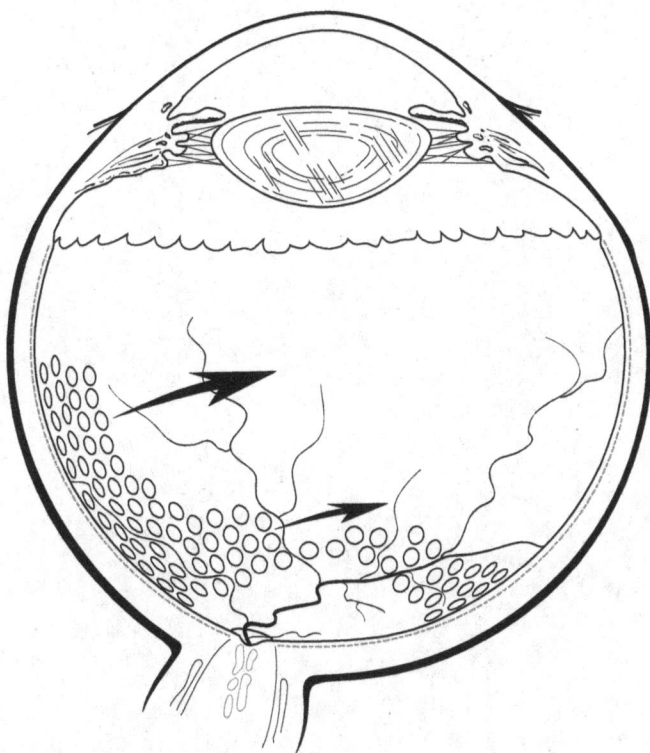

Figure 39-3

40

Focal Macular Photocoagulation

INDICATIONS

Diabetic macular edema; nonclearing macular edema secondary to vascular occlusive event; selected cases of central serous chorioretinopathy

EQUIPMENT

- Contact lens
- Topical anesthetic
- Coupling solution
- Argon laser

TECHNIQUE

1. Place a drop of topical anesthetic in the eye.
2. Place the contact lens of choice onto the selected eye with coupling solution. Ensure that there are no air bubbles.

3. Laser settings:
   - 50- to 100-μm spot size
   - Argon green wavelength
   - 0.1-second duration
   - 100 mW initial power
4. Treat leaking microaneurysms that are greater than 500 μm from the center of the macula directly with the focal laser. Grid laser treatment is applied to areas of diffuse edema. Burns should be no closer than one burn-width apart. Avoid placing spots in areas of hemorrhage (Fig. 40-1).
5. Adjust the power in small increments so that only a mild whitening of retina is seen.

PITFALLS

- Avoid placing spots in the foveal avascular zone.
- Possible side effects include paracentral scotomas, choroidal neovascularization, and scar expansion.

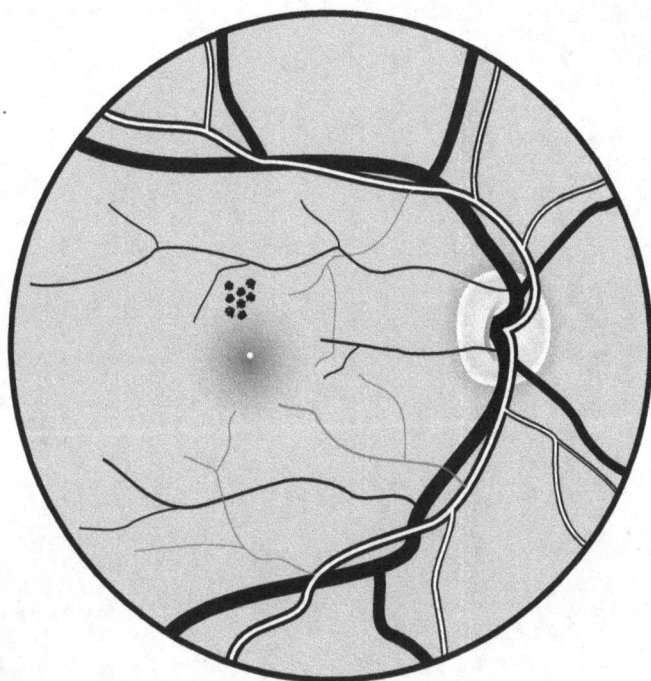

Figure 40-1

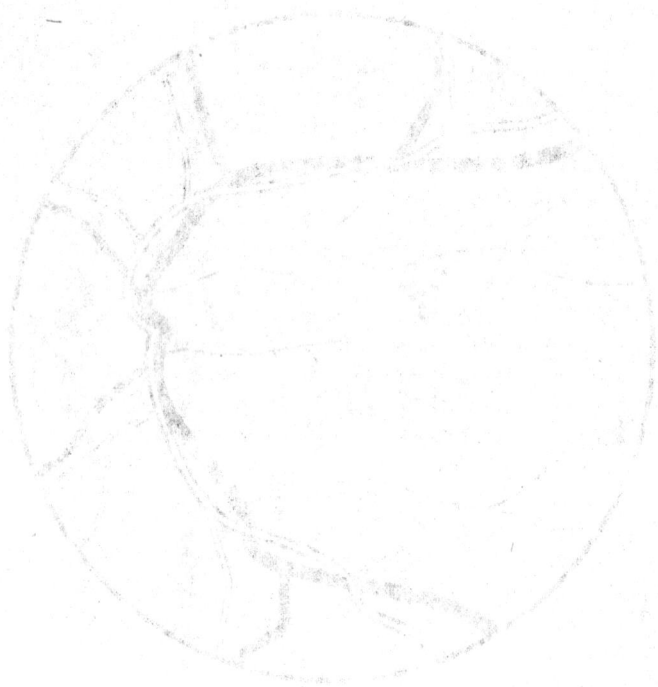

Appendix A

Common Ophthalmic Medications

Class	Drug	Brand name*	Route	Mechanism of Action	Side Effects
ANTIGLAUCOMA					
beta-blockers	betaxolol carteolol levobunolol metipranolol timolol	Betoptic Ocupress Betagan Optipranolol Timoptic, Betimol	drop drop drop drop drop	decreased aqueous production	exacerbation of asthma, bradycardia, fatigue, impotence, blunting of hypoglycemia in diabetics
beta-2-adrenergic agonists	apraclonidine brimonidine	Iopidine Alphagan	drop drop	decreased aqueous production	allergy tachyphylaxis
carbonic anhydrase inhibitors	acetazolamide dorzolamide methazolamide	Diamox Trusopt Neptazane	oral drop oral	decreased aqueous production	tingling in fingers and toes, dysgeusia, fatigue, GI upset metallic taste
osmotics	glycerin isosorbide	Osmoglyn	drop drop	dehydration of vitreous	exacerbation of CHF, fluid shifts
prostaglandin analogues	latanoprost travoprost bimatoprost unoprostone	Xalatan Travatan Lumigan Rescula	drop drop drop drop	increased uveoscleral outflow	darkening of iris color exacerbation of uveitis
sympathomimetics	epinephrine dipivefrin	Propine	drop drop	increased aqueous outflow	adrenochrome deposits, allergy epinephrine prodrug, allergy
direct acting cholinergic agents	carbachol pilocarpine	Isoptocarbachol Pilocar, Isoptocarpine	drop drop, gel	increased trabecular outflow	brow ache, retinal detachment, cataract formation
indirect-acting cholinergic agents	ecothiophate physostigmine	Eserine	drop ointment	increased trabecular outflow	brow ache, retinal detachment, cataract formation

ANTIBIOTICS

sulfonamides	sulfacetamide	Bleph-10	drop, ointment	interferes with bacterial synthesis of folic acid	allergy
	trimethoprim-polymyxin B	PolyTrim	drop		
fluoroquinolone	ciprofloxacin	Ciloxan	drop	interference with bacterial DNA gyrase	precipitation of drug on epithelial surface
	ofloxacin	Ocuflox	drop		
	levofloxacin	Quixin	drop		
	moxifloxacin	Vigamox	drop		
	gatifloxacin	Zymar	drop		
aminoglycoside	gentamicin	Gentak	drop, ointment	blocks protein synthesis	epithelial toxicity
	tobramycin	Tobrex	drop, ointment		
cell-wall active	vancomycin		drop, intravitreal	disruption of the cell wall	
macrolide	erythromycin		ointment	blocks protein synthesis	
	azithromycin	Zithromax	oral		
tetracyclines	tetracycline		ointment, oral	inhibit protein synthesis	
	doxycycline		oral		
	minocycline		oral		
miscellaneous	chloramphenicol		drop	inhibits protein synthesis	aplastic anemia
	bacitracin		ointment	inhibits cell wall synthesis	
	clindamycin		intravitreal	suppresses protein synthesis	
	polymyxin B		drop, ointment	disruption of the cell wall	

(Continued)

Class	Drug	Brand name*	Route	Mechanism of Action	Side Effects
ANTIFUNGALS					
polyene	amphotericin B		drop, intravitreal, IV	disrupts cell wall	renal toxicity with IV dosing
pyrimidine	flucytosine		oral	inhibits RNA synthesis	
imidazole	ketoconazole		oral	inhibits synthesis of ergosterol	
	miconazole		oral		
	clotrimazole		oral		
triazole	fluconazole		oral	inhibits fungal cytochrome P450	
ANTIVIRALS					
nucleoside analogue	trifluridine 0.1%	Viroptic	drop	interferes with viral DNA synthesis	
	idoxuridine 1%	Herplex	drop		
	vidarabine 3%	Vira-A	ointment		
	acyclovir	Zovirax	oral		
	famciclovir	Famvir	oral		
	valacyclovir	Valtrex	oral		
ANTIINFLAMMATORY					
corticosteroids (topical)	dexamethasone	Maxidex	drop	suppression of immune system	cataract formation
	fluorometholone	FML	drop		steroid-induced glaucoma
	prednisolone acetate	PredForte	drop		
	prednisolone phosphate	Inflamase Forte	drop		
	rimexolone	Vexol, Alrex	drop		
	loteprednol	Lotemax	drop		
non-steroidal antiinflammatory	ketorolac	Acular	drop	interruption of prostaglandin	
medication	diclofenac	Voltaren	drop	synthesis	
	flurbiprofen	Ocufen	drop		
	suprofen	Profenal	drop		

(Continued)

	Generic	Brand	Form	Mechanism	Toxicity
mast cell stabilizers	cromolyn sodium	Crolom	drop	stabilizes mast cell membranes	
	lodoxamide	Alomide	drop		
antihistamine	levocabastine	Livostin	drop	H1-specific antagonist	
	naphazoline	Naphcon, Vasocon	drop		
	nedocromil	Alocril	drop		
MYDRIATICS AND CYCLOPLEGICS					
alpha-adrenergic agonist	phenylephrine		drop		hypertension with 10% solution
parasympatholytics	atropine		drop		anticholinergic toxicity
	scopolamine	Hyoscine	drop		
	homatropine		drop		
	cyclopentolate	Cyclogyl	drop		
	tropicamide	Mydriacyl	drop		
alpha-adrenergic blocker	dapiprazole	Rev-Eyes	drop	reverses dilation of pupil	
ANESTHETICS					
	proparacaine	Alcaine	drop		epithelial toxicity
	tetracaine		drop		

* Many of these medications are available in a generic formulation. Other brand names may also be available and are not listed.
Note: There are many new drugs in the pipeline. Their use in the armamentarium of ophthalmology is yet to be established.

Appendix B

Basic Ophthalmic Instruments

For easier recognition and identification, illustrations of some of the surgical instruments which are useful for many ophthalmic procedures are shown below. Photographs courtesy of Storz Instruments (a division of Bausch & Lomb Surgical).

Lacrimal Kit

Lacrimal cannula

Punctal dilator

Bowman probes

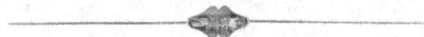

Pigtail probe

Chalazion Kit

Chalazion clamp

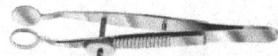

Chalazion curette

Fixation forceps

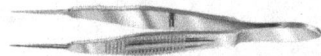

Westcott scissors

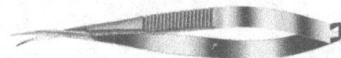

Plastics Kit

Bishop-Harmon toothed forceps

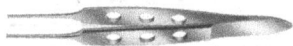

Castroviejo needle holder

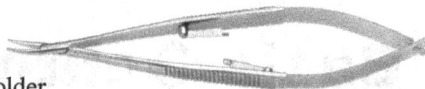

Suture scissors

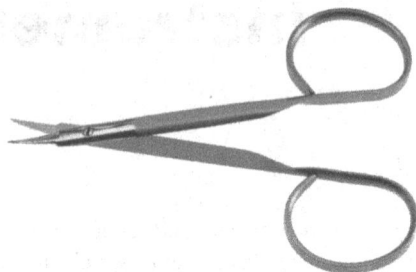

Index

Note: Page numbers followed by the letter "*t*" indicates tables; those followed by the letter "*f*" indicate figures.

www.ingramcontent.com/pod-product-compliance
Lightning Source LLC
Chambersburg PA
CBHW011225210326
41598CB00039B/7314